ART
as
MEDICINE

ALSO BY SHAUN McNIFF

Depth Psychology of Art (1989)
Fundamentals of Art Therapy (1988)
Educating the Creative Arts Therapist (1986)
The Arts and Psychotherapy (1981)

ART as MEDICINE

Creating a Therapy of the Imagination

SHAUN McNIFF

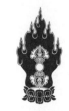

SHAMBHALA

Boston & London

1992

Shambhala Publications, Inc.
Horticultural Hall
300 Massachusetts Avenue
Boston, Massachusetts 02115

© 1992 by Shaun McNiff

9   8   7   6   5   4   3   2

Printed in the United States of America on acid-free paper
⊗
Distributed in the United States by Random House, Inc., and in
Canada by Random House of Canada Ltd

Library of Congress Cataloging-in-Publication Data
McNiff, Shaun.
Art as medicine: creating a therapy of the imagination / Shaun
McNiff.—1st ed.
p.   cm.
Includes bibliographical references and index.
ISBN 0-87773-658-8 (alk. paper)
1. Art therapy.   2. Creation (Literary, artistic, etc.)—
Therapeutic use.   3. Imagery (Psychology)—Therapeutic use.
4. Psychotherapy.   I. Title.
RC489.A7M356   1992   92-50117
615.8'5156—dc20   CIP

For Jack

Contents

Acknowledgments

In addition to my four children and my wife, Catherine Cobb, who has been a valued listener and critic, other supporters during the hatching of *Art as Medicine* include Vincent Ferrini in Gloucester; the spirit of Truman Nelson hovering over all of the Essex County coast; my faithful manuscript readers Paolo Knill and Margot Fuchs; Lesley College colleagues and graduate students; Helen Landgarten in Los Angeles and Jacqueline McAbery in San Francisco; Sr. Kathleen Burke and Bruce Moon in Ohio; Jerrilee Cain in Illinois; Lynn Kapitan and Lori Vance in Wisconsin; Bob Blumberg in Iowa; Steve and Ellen Levine in Toronto and Martha's Vineyard; Howard McConeghey in Albuquerque and the Southwestern College community in Sante Fe; Gunda Graenicher in Zurich; Majken Jacoby in Copenhagen; Baruch Zadick and the Arts Institute community in Tel Aviv; and James Hillman and Thomas Moore in the archetypal stream. Sincere thanks to Shambhala Publications and Kendra Crossen for giving me the opportunity to express *Art as Medicine* in the body of this book, and thanks to Lorraine Kisly for editing the manuscript.

ART
as
MEDICINE

Introduction

The soul is a very perfect judge of her own motions, if your mind does not dictate to her. . . . The soul's deepest will is to preserve its own integrity, against the mind and the whole mass of disintegrating forces.

Soul sympathizes with soul.

—D. H. LAWRENCE (1923)

WHENEVER ILLNESS is associated with loss of soul, the arts emerge spontaneously as remedies, soul medicine. Pairing art and medicine stimulates the creation of a discipline through which imagination treats itself and recycles its vitality back to daily living.

My perspective on medicine is artistic. I will not be making bioenergetic assessments of pulse beats altered by meditations on images. Although the chemistry of the body no doubt changes as a result of artistic expression and reflection, the purpose of this book is to engage them as modes of psychological inquiry. Rather than attempting to explain the artistic emanations of soul, our psychology desires to activate and move soul by striving to speak its own language.

The methods and philosophy in this book are based on principles of dialogue and interplay. Creation is interactive, and all of the players are instrumentalities of soul's instinctual process of ministering to itself. Conflict as well as affection propel the process.

Art as medicine does not restrict its interactions to human relationships. Concentration on the "other" ensouls the world, and paintings are ensouled objects or beings who guide, watch, and accompany their makers and the people who live with them. Their medicine is established by this "otherness," which enables them to influence people who open themselves to receiving help from another.

I intend this to be a practical book, based on life experiences, but not

1

limited to descriptions of those experiences. The book is itself a "doing," an action in which soul demonstrates how it moves within the individualized yet archetypal context of a person's life. The word *soul* suggests the essential nature of persons and other phenomena. It is characterized by individuality, the aesthetic quality, or aura, that distinguishes one thing from another. It is also an inner movement or stirring, the force of creative animation and vitality. *Soul* is closely related to and sometimes synonymous with *psyche, daimon,* and other words that appear frequently in this text. All of these words emanate from a common mystery. Their purpose is poetic rather than explanatory, and through them the soul experiences itself more deeply. Throughout the book I will use the word *image* and generally refer to the visual images of dreams and pictures, but movements, sounds, poetry, enactments, and ideas are not excluded from my sense of the word.

As soon as a painting is made, or a dream remembered, the images that constitute their being are experienced as wholly other. This autonomous life of the image is the foundation of a revolutionary and pragmatic treatment of our psychic diseases. We see the dogs, automobiles, houses, and rivers in our paintings and dreams as parts of ourselves, confirming the egocentric madness of our reality. Everything is reduced to the perspective of the experiencing "I."

It is through others that we discover who we are. When we learn how to step aside and watch ourselves, the other becomes an agent of transformation. Dialoguing with images is a method for expanding ego's singular vision. In opening to others, we do not have to give away our place within the interaction. Others have an experience of us that may be quite different from our experience of ourselves. All of these perspectives are elements in the psychic stew. Reality is an ever-changing interplay and never a single, fixed position.

The dialogue between an artist and a painting is rarely limited to "twofold" communication. Many figures within the painting and the artist enter these conversations. It becomes increasingly clear that the first-person perspective of the artist, the "I" who is speaking, is composed of varied voices. On entering the world of the painting, we become aware of the many who speak through us, not just the figures in the pictures, but also the varied aspects of our thought. The articulation of these diverse "persons" is yet another aspect of image dialogue.

Virtually every person who uses art in psychotherapy believes in the ability of the image to expand communication and offer insight outside the scope of the reasoning mind. However, there are sharp distinctions in how we treat pictures once they appear. These attitudes range from approaching them as graphic signs for evaluating the mental conditions of artists, to greeting them as angels who come to offer assistance.

I view the making of art as a medicine that proceeds through different phases of creation and reflection. Although therapists and other people involved in this process make their contributions as guides and witnesses, the medicinal agent is art itself, which releases and contains psyche's therapeutic forces. The medicine offered by meditation on art is generally an infusion of imagination and awareness rather than a specific answer. "Messages" may ultimately be less significant than the engagement of images. Rather than understanding the "meaning" of the dreamer's pleasurable slide down a long pole into the darkness, we enjoy the slide and hold on to the image.

Yet artistic images encourage us to look at them and reflect upon their natures, both physical and psychological. Interpretation enters the world of the image and responds to its nature. Rather than labeling pictures from our frames of reference, we meditate on them, tell stories about how we created them, speak to them, listen to what they have to say, dramatize them through our bodily movement, and dream about them. All of these methods are dedicated to the ongoing release of art's expressive medicine. Analysis and reason make many contributions to our meditations, but they do not dominate.

Interpretive dialogue offers artists a psychology that resonates with the shaping of images. Although our emphasis here is on the personal and intimate dialogue between individual painters and their pictures, the same principles can be applied to "public" art. Inner dialogue and meditation enable a person to establish a private relationship with any art object. This mode of interpretation can be likened to Henry Corbin's vision of "creative prayer" as an "intimate dialogue" between two beings who depend upon one another and whose interaction leads to "new creations."

Since every aspect of art contributes to its medicine, we do not assume that some expressions heal and others do not. Negative and disturbing images are vital stimulants for healing in that the toxin is the antitoxin. Art's medicine trusts spontaneous expression and avoids

prescriptions—bright colors to cure depression, heroic figures to con-
quer fear, good energies to overwhelm bad. The grotesqueness of
Bosch's underworld is welcomed together with the serenity of Monet's
water lilies. Creative expression of the soul's aberrations gives them
the opportunity to affirm rather than threaten life.

Paradoxically, it is the particulars of ordinary life that open to
archetypal existence. The only way to soul's authentic and firsthand
movement is through the medium of our most personal materials
endowed with archetypal significance. The fact that in this book I use
my own paintings to demonstrate interpretive dialogue may strike
some readers as a contradiction to my admonition against egoism. My
objective, though, is the demonstration of a *method* of relating to
images that will help reshape our relationship to art in and out of
therapy. It is the life of imagination that I hope to convey and not the
details of the artist's life.

Although I have published many dialogues with other people in
which we work with their art, I am not focusing on that aspect here. I
want to show how an artist dialogues with his own pictures and how
the many figures of imagination speak through the process. Direct
engagement of images will, I hope, be instructive for therapists interested in methods that they can use with their patients. My focus here is
on the engagement of the "persons" of the image. As Jung suggests, a
better understanding of inner processes will benefit what we do in the
"outer" world of therapeutic practice.

In using my own pictures, I can take risks, speak freely, and publish
the contents of intimate dialogue. I do not want to use another person's
private expression to elucidate my methods. And no doubt my commitment to the ethics of how we use images in therapy and psychology
shapes my methods. Only the total involvement of "expert" interpreters in every phase of the artistic process will protect images and
artists from those who claim authority in a realm they never visit.
Taking on the role of helper demands a continuous examination of
how I am living the process I encourage in others.

The provision of medicine for the body and soul is one of art's many
functions. Other aspects of art, and especially its importance as a
commodity and its role as an indicator of ephemeral tastes, have
dominated our culture and alienated us from the healing muses. Art
itself may be in need of treatment, and there is no stronger and more
reliable remedy than its eternal function as articulator of the soul's

uncensored purpose. This enduring role is performed by radically personal, risky, sometimes offensive, and intimate art works that embrace psychic spontaneity—rather than market planning or political approval—as the basis of creation. Artists as well as people in therapy ask for this medicine, and art is ready to respond when we establish the context for treatment. For over two decades my work has responded to this calling, and I see clearly that the fulfillment of the vision demands the dissolution of boundaries between the communities of the arts and healing. In those rare moments when the best resources of both are gathered in a shared commitment, we experience a satisfaction achieved only by the realization of "the soul's deepest will."

This book begins with a description of the varied influences that have shaped my experience of art as medicine. These reflections are followed by an attempt to examine the methodological essentials of interpretive dialogue, after which we return to the living sea of practice through meditations on images.

Part One

CONTEXT

Simple Beginnings

IN THE WINTER of 1970 I was a twenty-three-year-old law school dropout in Salem, Massachusetts, committing my life to art. A three-month job in an iron works at $2.25 an hour lost its appeal as soon as I learned how to weld steel. I had worked as a welfare caseworker in Brooklyn during the summer after college, so I found myself filling out a job application for social work at Danvers, the local state hospital. The personnel director looked at my application and told me that the hospital was only hiring social work graduates. He then added, "But with your background in painting, you might be interested in an art therapy position."

I had never heard of art therapy before and replied, "Can you say more about that?"

"We had an art student who worked here for a summer. She started an art program and continued with it for a while after graduating, but she's moved to Hawaii. Would you like to talk to the director of occupational therapy?"

"Sure."

The director of personnel had been in charge of volunteers for many years, and it happened that my grandmother was one of their mainstays. She did knitting and sewing with the patients at the hospital every Thursday for over twenty years, and during the summer she had garden parties for them at her house in Peabody. I helped her make vats of juice from her grape vines for the patients and their attendants.

Without having had time to think, I found myself sitting in the office of the director of occupational therapy, who asked, "What is your philosophy of art therapy and how would you put it to work here at the hospital?"

I said something about what the process of making art can do for people by engaging their senses in purposeful and gratifying activity,

and recall making a pitch for encouraging people to do things naturally and become involved in what they do.

The director did not care for projective confabulations about pictures being presented as facts about the artist's psyche, and so the issue
that has inspired my work for over two decades was also my entrance
into a career. Unwittingly selected by a philosophy, and by a woman
who apparently liked my practicality, I walked out of the hospital an
"art therapist."

One patient who had been in the institution for over thirty years
answered my question about how he was first admitted by saying, "I
was traveling around New England and I stopped to have a smoke
with a group of patients outside Worcester State Hospital and the
attendants took me back in with them and I have been inside ever
since." His story of how he became a patient is no less plausible than
my account of becoming an art therapist.

When I began to work as an art therapist, I sensed, but did not fully
understand, the medicine in the artistic process. I was too close to the
work to see what was happening, but it was clear that something
essential was missing in both medicine and art. Something was lost in
each as they moved away from one another through the course of our
culture's history. Today I still feel the loss of their aboriginal relationship and reciprocal caring for the soul.

In retrospect, my primary therapeutic and artistic advantage was
that I never belonged within the system. I was in an unfamiliar situation, so something had to be created from scratch. The world of art
offered only the individualistic and heroic model of the artist who
strives to generate a "reputation" and an industry of his person. There
were no divinity schools of creative expression, no organized communities of artists striving to serve society. In the medical/psychiatric
establishment every other discipline was adjunctive with professions
like psychology gradually moving up the hierarchy as the medical
doctors left public service. Instinct informed me that we were going
nowhere within the hierarchies. The artistic *daimon* of therapy took up
residence in me as a guide and suggested new combinations outside the
established routines of both mental health and art. The daimon (plural,
daimones) is an archetypal agent, creation itself, that speaks through us.

I mean no disrespect to colleagues in psychiatry, nursing, social
work, psychology, and the arts. To the contrary, I have always believed
that cooperation, honest disagreement, and consensus are essential

features of community life. But art is a medicine that can revolutionize therapy, and its transformative impact will be realized only if it continuously offers a radically different paradigm. The excessive reliance on chemical therapies, hierarchical control, and other institutional practices of "health" have to be looked at from a completely foreign perspective in order to be seen. Once art accommodates itself to these practices and becomes assimilated into the system, it no longer provides this perspective.

My daimon has always insisted on the undiluted use of artistic medicine. This orientation does not necessarily favor "art" over "therapy." Medical professions have been the ground upon which the work is practiced, and they have provided the forum for reflection upon philosophies, methods, and identity. I avoid conceptual opposition between therapy and art, preferring to follow the lead of the purposeful psyche, or guiding daimon, as it expresses needs to paint, perform, talk, reflect, or seek help.

Mental health and therapeutic services have attracted artists who desire to commit their lives to the care of soul. In our era the suffering soul finds itself in the clinic, and from history we will discover that revolutionary and spiritual transformations occur when soul exists *in extremis*. Pathology and wounds open us to the life of the soul.

More than twenty years after my first days in the hospital, I was invited as consultant to a large state hospital, where I watched the music therapist working with a woman who was composing original songs about her religious and sexual desires. I talked with a young man who, after looking through a book in the hospital library about William Blake, worked alone in his room producing a wondrous series of drawings. When the man was depressed and committed to a mental hospital, Blake appeared as a soul guide. This patient's drawings of animals, distorted faces, flying forms, and figures that combined animal and human qualities tapped into the same archetypal stream that flows through Blake's art.

When I began to work at Danvers, any picture that portrayed imaginative scenes and presented the inner movements of psyche was considered an expression of psychopathology. The conventional mind does not know how to see expressions of the chthonic and irrational soul as natural. "Health" is considered to be a faithful representation of a "reality" that also happens to fit the perceptual bias of the viewer. As a result of these conditions I immediately took on the role of protector of the images that emerged from outside that reality. I provided a safe and affirming place for their emergence and preservation. It was a *temenos*, a sacred precinct, where soul paintings covered the walls and welcomed those yet to come.

My work today with art as medicine outside the asylum context involves the creation of a sanctuary where people experience the process of caring for the soul through painting together, meditating collectively on the images, dialoguing with them, and making performances. Nothing has changed with regard to the substance of the work except that it is better known, and people choose to come. This attraction to art as medicine, and the openness people bring to the process, significantly deepens the experience and increases the powers of suggestion and persuasion that form the basis of every medicine.

In describing what we do, I frequently say, "The simpler, the deeper." Simplicity brings feelings of depth because it liberates us from the need to explain everything. A one-sided use of reason traps us in the intellect. I do not want to suggest that expression is simple. It is extraordinarily complex and unpredictable, but simple methods enable us to embrace complex contents and movements.

Although my art therapy studios are focused on painting, the graduate school of arts in psychotherapy that I started in 1973 places few limitations on the subject matter of artistic experience. Life itself is the material of art. Individual artists are encouraged to experiment and find styles and methods of expression that resonate with their natures and the needs of soul. Like shamans, therapists and patients alike open to the forces working within them through meditations and individual quests. I am sympathetic to the Zen monasteries, which encourage people to fully experience what they are doing when they eat, walk, or sit. When a beginner wants a list of directions, clinical ramifications, and a description of the theoretical approach, I say, "Paint."

The same orientation applies to dancing, writing, and other arts. I encourage "beginner's mind" and make the artistic process as simple as possible, describing how planned strategies block spontaneity. In order to operate within this context, the artist has to relax ego and see it as only one of many players within expression's pantheon. Curiosity and attentiveness become active participants in the creative process as we learn how to watch what we do while we are doing it. This is not easy, because our ego "judges" are thoroughly ingrained in us, but struggles abate as commitment and familiarity increase. Art becomes part of the tradition of meditation where watchfulness is essential.

Whatever a person paints, dances, or sings has significance when we restrain ego's value judgments. These discoveries are similar to the meditator's experience of wonder in something that was once boring and insignificant. Judgment yields to awareness.

So I am asked, "How do you make a painting better? Criticism is essential to art. How do you perfect the discipline?"

Through immersion in it. If you are able to watch and respond to thresholds that emerge in their time, the process offers unending depth, surprises, and challenges. Creation is a sentient and instinctual flow that determines where to go and what to change or omit.

The most fundamental and useful technique in this work is the ability to look at ego, the "I," as one of many players or collaborators in the creative process. This perspective on ourselves avoids complete identification with the feeling of the moment. We are able to look at fear, anger, desire, ecstasy, depression, success, failure, and other emotions as phenomena with which we interact. They move through us. Change is guaranteed only if I can let go of my attachment to each feeling as it appears. New Englanders say that if you don't like the weather, don't worry, because it will change. Expression is similarly characterized by fluctuations, while ego tends to lock onto things, especially things it does not like. It gets caught in a single point of view. Standing outside this perspective and observing it operate is the best medicine I know for psyche's ailments. Step aside and watch.

When I look at ego as one of many inner figures, I am amused by its actions. I observe its foibles with compassion and acceptance. Ego is not rejected, because it is a part of the process. Suppression only increases its power, whereas if I watch ego as a psychic figure, I am not completely possessed by it. Creative interaction and change replace possession and fixity.

When the harsh critic speaks up as you begin to paint and your insecurity and fear take hold, relax and observe. Look the intimidator in the eye and say, "Hello. It is time for us to talk. Let's get to know each other."

Artistic values affirm the individual's freedom of inquiry, and methods of practice will be as varied as people. I have been little more than a builder of the studio and a keeper of the artistic process that itself does the work of therapy. When beginning work with a group, my methods are simply the starting point, and are continuously transformed by the group.

The skill involved has to do with learning to help people relax, to watch the flow of painting from the soul, and to realize that their individual style will emerge. In addition to stimulating and inspiring expression, one needs to allow space for creation to express itself spontaneously and individually. Yet there is also a need for continued support and guidance through the phases of the experience, something I did intuitively during my first years at Danvers.

This way of working is radically different from technique-oriented systems of contemporary psychotherapies. Our therapeutic values affirm diversity and the vitality and wisdom of spontaneous expression realized through freedom of movement and a moment-to-moment appreciation for what is taking place.

The word *psychotherapy* is descriptive of art as medicine because we clearly operate within a context that attends to psyche. This is not an "art *as* therapy" orientation as opposed to "art *in* therapy." Polarizations limit the situation. The artistic process itself is the basis, as it is in all depth psychologies where psyche manifests itself in images. Art as medicine is more than a studio experience where we learn how to paint and experience therapeutic results. The spontaneous expressions of participants demonstrate that deep movements of psyche are made visible through paint. Art as medicine is therefore a depth psychology. An approach that welcomes the spontaneous visitations of expression is a new and very old *modus operandi* that transcends the categories of "art as therapy," "art in therapy," et cetera.

In the early 1970s I searched without success for a tradition that would help me to connect to the work of others. Depth psychology was associated with psychiatry, not art. Rather than protecting and furthering the emanations of psyche, all of the guilds were busy guarding and advancing themselves.

The psychiatric and psychological traditions of analyzing paintings and drawings on the basis of theories of psychopathology made as little sense then as they do now. I was amazed that eminent professionals could say that little boys who make pictures of lawnmowers suffer from castration fears and that girls who draw vacuum cleaners experience oral deprivation. As a young painter drawn into art therapy during a compassionate era when I dreamt of making contributions to the transformation of society, analyzing shirt buttons in a drawing as manifestations of psychosexual pathology offered little to the revolution.

It didn't do much for the patients either. They knew they were troubled, and there was little ambiguity about what the problem was.

They suffered from comprehensive cognitive, emotional, and social disintegration. The most logical course was the one taken by my grandmother in her efforts to treat them with dignity rather than repulsion. I tried to do this through the creative process.

Within the context of the hospital, soul was not simply lost; it was suffering, and suffering acutely. The anguish of the suffering soul made expression and transformation through the arts such an obvious mode of treatment that I wondered why it was not taking place continuously in all sections of the hospital milieu. Although there are occasional and distinguished exceptions, we have given over the care of the soul to medications, institutions, and a host of procedures that continuously undermine its dignity. The suffering soul, the basis of our Western religious traditions, has been abandoned.

I discovered the existence of other pioneering art therapists in the United States and foreign countries through the *Bulletin of Art Therapy* (later changed to the *American Journal of Art Therapy*), but most approaches of the time looked for the illness in expression, and I was concerned with its vitality. Rudolf Arnheim, known as the leading psychologist of art, answered a "long shot" letter I wrote from the hospital and agreed to advise my master's degree studies as I continued to work full-time. His work on art and visual perception was immensely useful in treating psychosis through art. We worked directly on reorganizing perceptual and cognitive disintegration through the process of making art, looking at it, and talking about it. We were treating disorders of imagination through the constructive workings of imagination. From the very beginning the work with images was phenomenological, social, and imaginative. We engaged people where they were, and introduced art to their lives. This orientation does not deny psychopathology and its presence in our expression. Art therapy's embrace of *pathos* can actually contribute to the revitalization of art, which flourishes when it opens to the troubles of the soul.

Shamanic Continuities

THE MOST SUPPORTIVE and exciting materials that I read as a beginning art therapist were published by Hans Prinzhorn and others during Europe's Dada-Surrealist era, when artists were keenly interested in "outsider art." Prinzhorn (1972), writing in 1922, felt that the spontaneous art works of mental patients were "the eruptions of a universal human creative urge." This was in keeping with the life-affirming qualities I observed in the artistic expressions of the patients with whom I was working. Prinzhorn felt that the patients' art was a natural antidote to schizophrenic disintegration and alienation. From the autistic condition of psychosis, wondrous images emerged to accompany and guide the soul.

Prinzhorn, an art historian who later trained as a psychiatrist, was not interested in the intentional clinical use of the art works for diagnosis and treatment. He shared the Surrealists' sense of wonder in response to the manifestations of psyche, and suggested that the suffering soul should have access to the vital and natural medicine of art and imagination. Because of his lack of attention to a scientific use of art, Prinzhorn has not had a significant impact on the art therapy field. He was more interested in what art did than in the methods of therapists.

However, when we shift the perspective of art as medicine away from scientism to the treatment of soul, Prinzhorn becomes strikingly relevant. He proves that when the soul is lost, art comes spontaneously to its assistance. When the soul is depressed, isolated, mad, and distraught, artistic images appear. Prinzhorn noted, and we observed at Danvers, that people without a background in art began to create in response to their suffering. The creative imagination acts spontaneously as its own savior. When the intensity of the emotional unrest subsided, so did the art.

Prinzhorn was concerned with the universal implications of the soul's efforts to redeem itself. He made parallels between the asylum artists and the avant-garde themes of expressionism, basing his thought in Nietzsche's vitalism and a respect for the wisdom of instinctual expression. His belief that animals can teach us how to live naturally with our inner drives and environments corresponded to the psychology of D. H. Lawrence. He translated Lawrence's *The Man Who Died* into German, and in his book *Psychotherapy: Its Nature, Assumptions and Limitations* (1932) he said that the character and life experience of the therapist are the most essential factors and that writers are often more perceptive than psychologists.

Like Lawrence, Prinzhorn felt that excessive rationalism has alienated the soul from nature. C. G. Jung, expressing a similar sentiment, said that God was upset because man loved his reason more than "Him." Schizophrenia was not just a personal disease but a malady afflicting a civilization disconnected from its sources. Creative expression is a spontaneous and unconscious effort of the soul to treat itself in keeping with a "uniform metaphysical instinct." Prinzhorn affirmed this instinct and its expression by his patients, who, he said, are "in contact, in a totally irrational way, with the most profound truths, and have produced, unconsciously, pictures of transcendence as they perceive it" (1972, p. 242). Psyche expressed itself naturally through the art of these mental patients, which emerged without being influenced by academic and social conventions.

Prinzhorn's research was in keeping with my vision of art therapy, also guided by Nietzsche and Lawrence, as a return to the shamanic origins of art as medicine. Images and the artistic process are the shamans and familiar spirits who come to help people regain the lost soul. The emotionally disturbed persons that Prinzhorn studied demonstrate a shamanic instinct that flows through all of us. The extraordinary art made by people suffering from psychosis affirms that soulful paintings emerge when the person "lets go" of the controlling mind. Without romanticizing psychosis and the way it disturbs thought, we can say that those suffering from emotional upheavals are in direct contact with powerful energies that can be channeled into paintings. Of course, we do not have to be psychotic in order to paint from the soul, but the depth of an art work certainly corresponds to the psychic environment in which it is created. Artists typically have more direct and visceral contact with a realm that is available to every person, but Prinzhorn described how the "customs" and "rules" of social life keep most of us insulated from the expression of these archaic forces. He felt, nonetheless, that we are "metaphysically attuned to laws of existence, not realistically attuned to external facts" (1972, p. 242) and that an "ancient symbolism" exists in each of us.

In the mid-1970s I began to think of the creative arts therapies as contemporary manifestations of ancient shamanic continuities. I observed that the things we did in art therapy, and the images we made, resembled the rituals and artifacts of shamanism. We were unconsciously participating in the shamanic tradition, and as an art therapist who had difficulty calling himself an art therapist because of the profession's identification with "adjunctive therapies," I found parallels to shamanism appealing. Nothing seemed more primary than the tradition of the shaman. I realized that it was possible to be "metaphysically attuned" to the patterns and movements of expression without literally calling oneself a shaman. Actually, it is probably irrelevant what therapists call themselves. The label is far less significant than the contents of practice and attunement to the nameless movements of soul.

The image of the shaman, however, is useful as a guide to the archetypal nature of art as medicine. Psychic illness is an alienation of soul and a possession of the psyche by preoccupations, obsessions, fears, anxieties, and other distractive conditions that are contemporary equivalents of the aboriginal "evil spirits." The archaic medicine of the shaman draws out the deleterious elements from the body and revives soul.

As the "estranged" archetypal figure of the shaman appears spontaneously within the imagination of our world, it is taken literally by many people as a primitive psychopomp who threatens the "advances" of medical technology. Contemporary indigenous healers frequently cooperate with the medical profession. They see their services as complementary, and the same applies to the "inner" shamans who help us ensoul the environments and the machines with which we live.

When the soul is in the process of ministering to itself, shamans and other imaginal persons appear and converge in a process that I call art as medicine. My work also identifies with a tradition of artists who have committed their lives to art's regenerative and redemptive aspects in the personal, social, and spiritual spheres. Even revolutionary art is compatible with this transformative genre.

Art therapy can take us into the primary sources of sacred and psychological experience if we allow the shamans and spirits to emerge once again from images and imagination. Our contemporary fascination with shamanism is an expression of a hunger for experiences that engage and sanctify the total spectrum of life, and not just the human dimension. The shamanic perspective affirms the archetypal nature of the primal expressions in the pictures, dances, sounds, and dramas emerging from our art therapy studios.

The poetic or imaginal figure of the shaman is not necessarily in opposition to the literal shaman who practices in the world. However, exclusive reference to the shaman as a person who operates within foreign, distant, and inaccessible cultures guarantees that we will continue to imagine shamanic possibilities as foreign, distant, and inaccessible. The literal shaman who exists within indigenous communities can be imagined as the shamanic daimon beckoning us to search the native culture of personal expression.

Mircea Eliade said that "the shaman is indispensable in any ceremony that concerns the experiences of the human soul" (1964, p. 182). Therefore, it is natural for the shaman, always concerned with the welfare of soul, to appear when the psyche is in need. Soul's tradition of ministering to itself appeared spontaneously as I was searching for alignment with a depth psychology.

It might be asked: Does soul minister to itself, or does a guide, psychopomp, or shamanic archetype care for the soul?

Both, I reply. The inner shaman is a figure within the soul, one of its many aspects, which contribute to its well-being.

Shamanic images and patterns emerge whenever we engage ourselves in the therapeutic rituals of the arts in painting, dance, drama, song, and other media. Imagination has always been the terrain of shamans. Encounters with animals, openings into different worlds, dreamlike flights, and various other shamanic themes, artifacts, and experiences appear during rhythmic drumming, movement, chant, and painting. These images arrive whenever the soul opens to itself. There does not have to be a conscious involvement with "shamanism," since the images emerge autonomously, again affirming the soul's instinctual process of caring for itself.

James Hillman has referred to the image as "a *psychopompos*, a guide with a soul" (1983, p. 62). Perhaps the psychic image is the shaman that human beings imitate. This would account for the consistent presence of the shaman across cultures and the historical spectrum. In a culture such as ours, where there are no longer shamans operating with the full support of communities, shamanic figures will appear in dreams, meditations, art works, and rituals such as psychotherapy.

In addition to losing the shaman, we have lost our sensibility to the psychic figures, or images, that are always accessible as ways of reviving the shaman's ubiquitous commitment to soul. As a psychic figure, the shaman is a daimonic functionary, an intermediary who operates within the realm of imagination.

The notion of the shaman as a psychic figure who attends to soul fits Jane Harrison's definition of the daimon as a functionary rather than an individual person: "The *daimon* proper . . . was a collective representation expressing not a personality so much as a function" (1962, p. 315). This archetypal perspective helps us to look beyond personal histories and allows us to revise art history in terms of psychic functions. Rather than simply accept conventional concepts of what artists were doing during a particular epoch, we can follow Prinzhorn's advice and see art as "metaphysically attuned to laws of existence, not realistically attuned to external facts." This view does not require rejection of "external facts" and ordinary things on which we bestow archetypal significance.

Although there are many artists who illustrate the shamanic aspects of the creative process, few people in the twentieth century can parallel the commitment of D. H. Lawrence to the redaimonization of the world, to saving soul, through the medicine of art. Lawrence felt *mana* (divine power) in all things, all life. In *St. Mawr*, Cartwright described how Pan was once a "Great God," a "hidden mystery," before the Greeks gave him a distinct form: "I should say he was the God that is hidden in everything. In those days you saw the thing, you never saw the God in it: I mean in the tree or the fountain or the animal" (Lawrence, 1953, p. 54). Lawrence's entire opus is concerned with the salvation of soul, and, while he never spoke of himself as a shaman, he illustrates how the tradition functions outside human awareness. The artist's self-definition is in this respect superseded by the function of what he did and what the art does. Lawrence gives us a definition of art therapy when he says that "every true artist is the salvation of every other" when he or she becomes what he called "transmitters of life." The fact that Lawrence had no conscious relationship to art therapy or shamanism strengthens the archetypal significance of his work. It is the processes themselves that carry the shamanic lineage throughout the ages. As Lawrence said, "Never trust the artist. Trust the tale." Recognize and respect the forces that operate outside the scope of a single mind, epoch, or professional framework. These eternities communicate to us in ways that may have a "far deeper reference" than the artist imagined.

Shamanic cultures throughout the world describe illness as a loss of soul. The shaman's task is to go on a journey in the search of the abducted or lost soul and return it to the sick person. These "soul catchers" have been known to attach hooks to their fingers in order to hold on to souls.

Lawrence imagined Western civilization as sick and dying. His art is restorative. He is the archetypal soul searcher who realizes that expression is an endless pursuit of the "indefinite" deity.

The shamanic notion of soul loss is a metaphor for soul's tendency to elude the grasp of consciousness as well as its more primal detachment from feelings. The soul cannot be lost in a literal sense because it is always present with us. However, we do lose contact with its movements within our daily lives, and this loss of relationship results in bodily and mental illness, rigidification, the absence of passion, and the estrangement from nature. It is the nature of soul to be lost to that aspect of mind that strives to control it. Mind has to dissolve, to let go of its control, in order to experience what is not itself. Soul is a constant yet ephemeral motion that passes through us without containment. The loss of soul is a necessary element of our work, a prerequisite, because its absence stimulates a longing for its return. The experience of soul is a fleeting sensation of consciousness, and never a permanent or fixed condition.

The artist finds deep satisfaction through creative *kinesis* with its accompanying feelings of vitality and potentiality. For Lawrence this potency is the divinity, something he has called "vital energy," "soul," "the quick," "the unconscious." He preferred continuous and spontaneous movement to the containment of the daimon in fixed principles. For Lawrence, soul was lost when "pure relations" did not exist between himself and "the timber I am sawing . . . the dough I knead for bread." He said, "This is how I 'save my soul.' "

The salvation of soul comes when people engage their environment. Depth is in the textures, colors, and movements of actual things. Soul is missed and lost when we overlook the immediate presentation and try to determine what is behind or under it. Reflection on "hidden" meanings exercises the imagination of interpreters, but this pursuit cannot abandon the physical presence of the image.

Art as medicine embraces life as its subject matter, and separations among the arts are contratherapeutic. As I work with individuals, I am open to their poetic speech, stories, body movements, dramatic enactments, sounds, and other expressions as well as to the pictures they paint. I try to establish contact with as many aspects of the person's presence as possible.

All of the arts emerged naturally in my early creative arts therapy work with adults and children. Every art form is a dramatic enactment. Stories are constantly being told, bodies are always in motion. Experimentation with Paolo Knill and other colleagues during the 1970s revealed that shamanic enactments were impossible without the complete spectrum of artistic expression—drumming, movement, the use of images and objects, costuming, masks, and so forth. The novelist Truman Nelson, who worked with us during that period, spoke of how soulful expression is "chordal" as contrasted to "single-octave" sound. Norma Canner, our dance therapist in the multi-arts therapy program at Lesley College, focused on the natural expressions that every body makes. She discouraged recorded music and explored making sounds with instruments and the voice in response to movement rather than always dancing *to* the music. All of the arts were interacting with one another—poetry, painting, video, psychodrama and theater, music, dance, and storytelling.

Experience with art materials helped us to see how the flourishing imagination embraces diverse faculties. We learned how to follow expression in its varied movements. We similarly discovered how the affirmation of a group's diversity furthered the vitality of individual expression. Creativity is a contagious force.

History affirms the value of collaboration in the artistic process. Our stereotypic fantasy of the individual artist, creating alone and outside society, ignores art's history of cooperation and communal influences. To the extent that the work of the artist corresponds to the movements of soul in the world, the alienated artist is an expression of a contemporary malady. The artist who takes on the heroic values of our civilization lives out their tragic and unfulfilling consequences for all of us to witness, and reaffirms the need for community.

Art as medicine is a post-heroic phase in art's history. The way in which my work with others has taken place in group studios is yet another unplanned correspondence with the shamanic archetype. Individual heroics are replaced by the individuation of expression within a group that supports each member's natural and spontaneous emanation. A shamanic revival depends upon a believing community, and that support can come from a small and committed group of artists. The shamanic community of creation is in our genes waiting to be released.

Rather than teaching people through complicated procedures and techniques, my training groups in art therapy demonstrate how we can gain access to unrealized potentialities. While expression is inherently purposeful, creativity cannot be planned. For this reason, I am not comfortable assigning the subject matter of another person's art. In my studios I establish a clear structure and dependable rituals in terms of time, materials, and commitment to making and reflecting upon images, but we do not predetermine the nature of the images or the way in which a group should interact with them. Old philosophical ideas of "will" and "intention" are recast as a person's dedication and responsiveness to what appears spontaneously. Group leaders may march participants through established steps because they fear chaos and want to protect against it. They are surprised to discover that only the most elementary procedures of creation need to be established in advance.

Painters influence and stimulate one another with their images like musicians improvising with related sounds. Participants become what the Romantic poets called "agencies of the flying sparks." Soul moves about through charges and countercharges. I have observed that the studio of collaborative creation does not in any way restrict the particular styles and thematic concerns of individual artists. On the contrary, the absence of a single bias toward the values of painting gives each person the freedom to engage whatever emerges in a style which embraces soul's varied expressions.

Throughout my career I have followed the work itself. Using our multi-arts experimentation at Lesley as a basis, I gradually opened myself to new ways of practicing art therapy. Drumming and other percussive instruments were introduced to summon images and support their emergence. The drums help us to imagine painting as dance and movement. When we talk about pictures, our circle of painters is transformed into a community of storytellers. In response to the inspiration of performance artists, we began to interpret art through performance, the body, movement, and sound. Performance is not more advanced or "deeper" than talking, it is just different, another mode of communicating through which art therapy leads to *Gesamtkunstwerk* (Richard Wagner's term for total art work) and the full use of all artistic faculties. We respond to the images and gestures of a painting by presenting our bodies as images and gestures. At the same time, we maintain the discipline and tradition of the painting studio. The other arts enhance rather than dilute the making of pictures. Art itself benefits from a community of creation that involves different art forms and incites imagination through diversity. Collective involvement is yet another shamanic element that survives to manifest itself in every aspect of art as medicine.

Archaic medicine views pathologies as aspects of the soul's existence and illness as inhabitation by spirits. Since curses may be "brushed off," the person is seen as separate from the malevolent force inhabiting the body. Troublesome spirits can potentially visit anyone and daily life involves rituals of propitiation and protection. Pathologies are vital participants in the imagination of individual and community life. Their existence is not restricted to a designated group of sick persons who function as scapegoats for the community. There is an ongoing ecology of imaginal functions within the shamanic context.

Art as medicine revives archaic attitudes toward the pathologies that have always fueled expression. Creative arts therapists were originally drawn to use the arts in the treatment of mental illness, and this social mission is still fundamental to our identity. However, as we began to experiment among ourselves, we discovered that the therapeutic process of group creation had a profound impact on supposedly "healthy" people. No doubt we entered this work of helping others through creation because we felt a corresponding need within ourselves. The lost and suffering soul that we encounter within mental institutions is an aspect of our collective human nature, which calls for attention through the extreme conditions of psychopathology. Compassion and identification with these conditions is of course helpful to our patients, but the patients have also helped us, and they have helped the soul, by drawing our attention to its needs. When therapy confines itself to treating "sick people," its perspective is always of sickness. There is no opportunity for the pathology to have a productive interplay with other aspects of life, as we see in shamanic cultures.

James Hillman helped me to see how my insistence that art therapy works with the "healthy" and "nonpathological" aspects of the person was a reaction to models of therapy that classify people according to pathologies. The classifying mind has used pathology to further its schemes. Rather than seeing pathology in a painting or dream as something sick and negative, we can embrace it as part of the soul's nature. This orientation does not take us away from the clinic, the hospital, and the prison but instead deepens our therapeutic identification with those places where the soul's suffering is most extreme. Most important, we have discovered that psychopathology is not merely something to be cured by well-meaning professionals and therapeutic technologies. This attitude assumes the wellness of the helper and the sickness of the patient, and anyone who has spent time in a mental hospital as a patient or staff member knows that this is not the case. It is widely acknowledged that the therapeutic system is itself often pathological, and the staff find solace and a sense of purpose in their relationships with patients. When staff begin to openly accept the pathology of their interactions with one another, then the system is ready for transformation.

Therefore, pathology is not limited to patients. It is in all of us, a fundamental element of the soul. Those acutely afflicted by these pathologies need help, but there is a missing element in our therapies today. Tribal societies knew how to make use of those who were possessed by emotional upheavals. We do not. By trying to fix them, improve them, eliminate them, drug them, and cure them, we are showing that we have not grasped how they can help us. The best medicine I can offer to a troubled person is a sense of purpose, the feeling that what he is going through may contribute to the vitality of the community. The process is reciprocal.

My experiences with the extremes of psychopathology have taught me that the therapy of soul extends to every life situation. The shrieks of the mental hospital have made me aware of the stoic yet equally needy souls in every community. By working with the soul in cases of extreme pathology, therapists get to know the range and depth of its expressions and afflictions. But pathology is part of the terrain in every life, so why not embrace it as essential to the ecosystem of soul? Rather than undertaking the impossible task of eliminating my pathologies, I get to know them better and minimize their unconscious and harmful expression. It is not just "my" pathology that I encounter, but the pathology of the soul. The concept of therapy is transformed by viewing the efforts of patients and therapists as expressions of the soul's process of ministering to itself. All of us, in the varied roles we play both as helpers and as recipients of care, are involved with a common purpose. We are attracted to a sense of psychology and therapy that "moves" the soul. These values are quite different from psychological notions of explaining, controlling, and predicting, none of which are intended to activate the resources of soul.

Art as medicine returns the treatment of pathologies to ritual activities within the context of a sympathetic community. If soul's existence is inseparable from its pathologies, to restrict its exploration to hospitals and clinics restricts soul itself. By detaching pathology from an exclusive reference to sick persons, the therapeutic consciousness is let loose on every aspect of society. As soul thrives, everything around it thrives as well.

Embracing the soul's debased expression as expressed in the images of art and dreams involves a shift in consciousness that transforms psychotherapeutic values. I become more interested in acknowledging and feeling the condition than in "fixing" it. The exclusive believe that therapy repairs what is wrong keeps us in a condition of eliminating symptoms. When these attitudes are applied to psychic images, we essentially eradicate the expressions of soul rather than entertain them. I have learned to view art's pathological manifestations as "angels of the wound" who open us to the life of soul. The wounded animal that comes in a dream helps me to see soul's suffering as expressed in its language of imagery. The artist in my studio who paints distorted and shriveled humans, sometimes dismembered and expressing anguish, is not to be taken literally as a person who wants to do this to himself or to others. The paintings do not necessarily mean that he feels this way about himself, or that he has to work on his body. However, they do express an archetypal condition of soul. The images may be concerned with helping the artist express the suffering of the soul and his personal anguish. The paintings may help him to accept and care for feelings of vulnerability and fragmentation that live in the shadows of the "intact" ego.

The rejected image in a painting or dream is usually the one that has the most to offer. It opens to the unrealized spectrum of the soul's compassion.

Attunement to the Archetypal

ART AS MEDICINE is a preexisting process, what Prinzhorn described as a "metaphysical instinct." Rather than inventing methods, I try to allow the archetypal process of art therapy to reveal itself. I will describe a series of phases that I have gone through to illustrate this adaptation.

After making hundreds of simplistic sketches of the same house with a Christmas tree in front of it, Christopher, who had been in the hospital for thirty-five years, began to copy the design of his packet of *Bugler* tobacco (see page 28). He not only grasped the gestalt of the image, but he rendered it with an intriguing style. I encouraged him to imitate paintings by Picasso and other prominent painters, and he responded with original interpretations. I coached him with occasional technical advice, and he went on to draw pictures of people in the studio and a series of self-portraits (page 29). Through the seven years that we worked together, the quality of the work was maintained. I sometimes organized exhibitions during that period, and one of Christopher's shows at the School of the Museum of Fine Arts was selected by the *Boston Globe* art critic as one of his favorite small exhibits for the year of 1974.

Anthony was thirty-five when we began our work together. For twenty years he had lived in a locked ward without carrying on a conversation with another person. It was thought that he was severely retarded. After months of making the same scribble of a human figure, he began to draw objects and people in his environment in an original style (see page 30). With constant attention and support, he gradually spoke to me, touching his throat to feel the unfamiliar vibrations of dormant vocal chords.

Both Anthony and Christopher ultimately left the hospital, and their involvement with art ended without the supportive environment of a studio tailored to their needs.

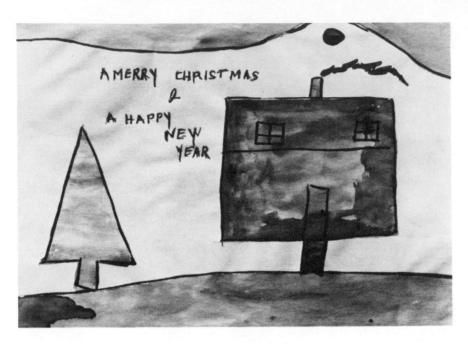

Christopher's early drawings.

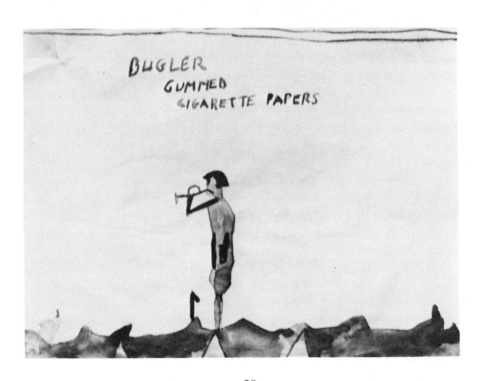

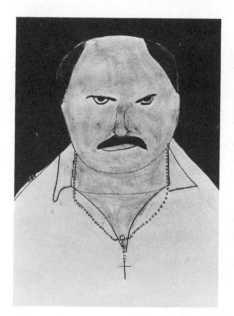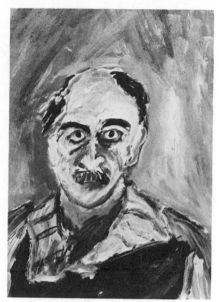

Christopher's later portraits.

As a young art therapist intent upon "proving" the therapeutic validity of my profession, I lectured about the "progress" of patients such as Christopher and Anthony and wrote papers about how "development" in art brings about corresponding changes in the person. But later I realized that my developmental model was constructed in response to the prevailing standards of the mental health world. The stories I told about Anthony and Christopher were really about the emotional impact those men, their pictures, and our studio environment were having on my life. I am not suggesting that the descriptions of my experience with Anthony and Christopher, presented in *The Arts and Psychotherapy* (1981), need to be revised, however. They have a detail of observation that I could not give today and there was a truthfulness to my sincere interest in their well-being.

Among the many people whom I saw in art therapy at that time was Priscilla, who introduced me to art as medicine. She had been living in institutions since her childhood and had been making fascinating art works years before I met her. Priscilla's paintings did not fit into the development theory I was constructing, but she was always eager to discuss her work, and she thrived on the community environment

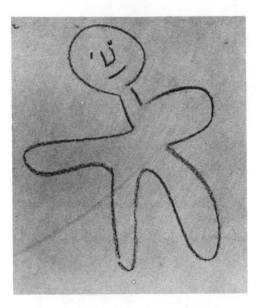

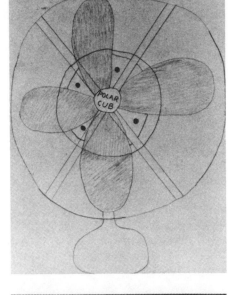

Anthony's art progressed from
scribbled figures to highly
original drawings.

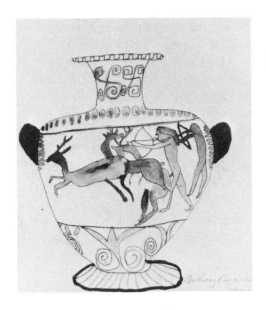

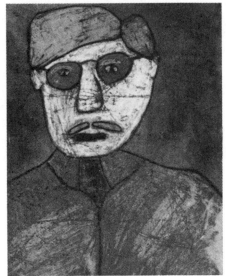

30

within our studio. Prior to the creation of the art therapy program, she worked in isolation and had accumulated hundreds of pictures and tin foil sculptures that were piled under a bed in the ward where she slept with sixty other women. In contrast to Christopher and Anthony, Priscilla, even when she painted scenes of people and places within the hospital, transformed them into an evocative expression of imagination (see below and page 32).

I see now that my time with Christopher, Anthony, and Priscilla probably had a far greater impact on my life than on theirs. Although I was the professional charged with helping them, and I assiduously addressed myself to that responsibility, they changed me. Their art inspired and changed my art. These three people affirmed the value of the work I was doing in art therapy. They became my guides and familiars. Whenever I talked about art therapy, I would give detailed accounts of what we did together.

After studying painting in New York City during the 1960s, I was a

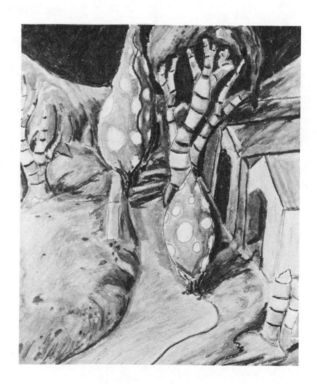

Priscilla's painting
of the hospital grounds.

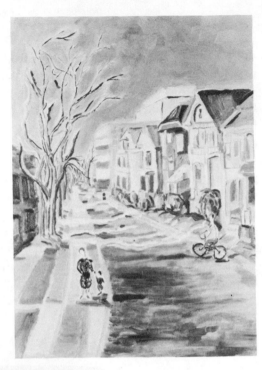

Priscilla's city street scene.

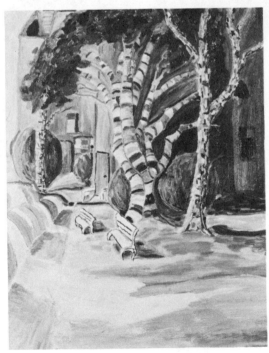

*Priscilla's painting
of the hospital grounds.*

devoted Abstract Expressionist. But within the environment of the hospital studio, it was ridiculous to talk about pure formal relations, minimalism, and the interactions of color. I did not bring my paintings to the art therapy studio, because I sensed that they were expressions from another world.

People asked me, "What do you paint? Aren't you going to show us your pictures?" Whenever I tried to explain, it was evident that we did not have a common frame of reference. On an instinctual level I realized that my art was an expression of a foreign culture, formalistic studies that lacked the visceral and direct passion of the paintings being made in the art therapy studio. At that time, I felt that I had to paint within the prevailing values of the "art world." I had not realized that the galleries I admired, and with which I longed to be involved, were often presenting a contrived and highly packaged form of art. I did not know it at the time, but my art education was being furthered by the archaic images that emerged naturally from the psyches of untrained painters within a mental hospital. As I helped patients to perfect their natural styles of expression, and as I worked with them in solving the structural problems presented by their pictures, I was being introduced to the primary process of painting and simultaneously educating myself without knowing what these collaborations would do to my life. I learned by watching, and the patients taught me the simple lessons of painting in a natural style. I observed that the expressive strokes of my handwriting and body movements were not present in my paintings. I realized that I could let a style of painting emerge that corresponded with my idiosyncratic ways of moving. I learned these lessons gradually and unconsciously, with no direct confrontation with my "New York" values, in the most unlikely environment for the training of an artist.

Today in art therapy, whenever people ask me how to begin, I say: "Just paint. Begin to move with the brush in different ways. Watch what comes. If you paint, it 'will come.' Nothing will happen unless you begin to paint, in your own way. Start painting as though you are dancing with your whole body, and not just using your fingers and your wrist. Use your arms with the force of the body behind them. Look at the shapes that appear, and think about what you can do with them."

This philosophy of creative expression is carved out of my experience and observations of the people with whom I have worked. The beginning painter often tries to represent images visualized in the mind in advance, making failure inevitable. It is virtually impossible for the beginner to render a replica of a mental image, and so the process becomes tight. I try to help people approach painting as tactile and movement-based. We deemphasize the "visual" dimension at first, to avoid concentrating too much attention in the controlling mind. In our first pictures we simply move and express feelings while trying to suspend criticism.

The method has always helped me as a painter when I begin to fall into fussy and habitual patterns of expression. Then the critical mind can enter the process as a "responsive" faculty that meditates on the image and shapes spontaneous gestures. In our studios we try to help painters establish this orientation to the "responding" mind rather than the "strategic planning" mind. The artistic consciousness seldom operates according to blueprints and roadmaps.

Nothing will happen unless a person begins and risks failure. And there will be constant failures and restarts and changes of direction along the way, all of which are essential to the emergence of something fresh and surprising. The same thing applies in the other arts. Nothing happens in the creation of a poem until the person starts to write. Ideas emerge from the movement of the hands and their interaction with the mind. All of the senses must collaborate if expression is to achieve psychic authenticity.

In the summer of 1968 after graduating from college, I was in New York making large minimalist paintings with stripes. As the paintings progressed to a series with one stripe across the surface, I concluded that the only way to go further with this vision of art was to stop painting altogether. Two years later the stripes came back in my paintings as an art therapist, but they were accompanied by fiery shapes and the canvas was no longer simply a flat, two-dimensional space. Strong feelings emerged through the pictures, but they were still intentional and conceptual efforts to link up with New York.

At that time I was in Salem working as an art therapist in the underworld of a state hospital, and I kept imagining myself in New York. Creation, like the dream, is shaped from the substance of daily life. Like it or not, I was emerging from a humble "art therapy school of painting," located in a grimy state hospital.

I was afraid to expose my artistic inadequacies when I was working with people as "their" art therapist. It was not until I left my job at the hospital that I went back to paint together with the patients. I wanted to make pictures of the people and their environment. My trips back to the hospital affirmed how the context was shaping my expression.

It is the movement through life that allows the artist's inner nature to emerge into an authentic style. Plans and ambitions have to give way and follow the soul as it moves through the local environment. Images come to us through the simple events of daily life. As D. H. Lawrence said in *Fantasia of the Unconscious*, "Learn to walk in the sweetness of the possession of your own soul" (1986, p. 147). Over and over again I discover and rediscover how it is the unlikely and difficult aspects of a person's life that fuel creation.

"Creative blocks" usually result from expectations that take us away from our immediate experiences. When art therapists ask me how I deal with blocks to expression, I talk to them about how important it is to engage the context of our present life and let the art flow from that source. I create from where I am and not from where I think I should be.

Art that I have made over the past two decades has increased my understanding of the art therapy process. The first direct link between art therapy and personal expression came in response to the difficulties generated by daily life.

I bought a large old house at the beginning of an oil crisis. It had been a summer house for over seventy-five years, and there was no insulation. We moved in the fall and had a few weeks to insulate. Installing fiberglass in tight and unventilated crawl spaces was a horrible job. When I put my foot through a ceiling, I really became depressed. It occurred to me that if I was preaching the merits of art therapy, I must apply it to myself. Until this point, art therapy had been completely separate from my personal life and art.

I photographed the rolls of insulation, the tools I used, the house, the hole in the ceiling—and began to view the project as a work of art. This shift of perspective, from drudgery to aesthetics, transformed my feelings. I started to enjoy the work, and I even dismantled parts of the job to take comprehensive "before" and "after" photos. The experience taught me about art's alchemical power to transform irritation into delight. I was creating directly from my daily life, from my anxiety.

Soon after the insulation project, my job as the dean of a graduate program was turning into a routine of meetings. In addition to meetings at the college, I was on the executive board of the American Art Therapy Association and active in other national organizations. Life was a series of all-day meetings in soulless hotel conference rooms without windows. I longed for fresh air, more contact with nature, and liberation from meeting rooms and offices. Yet I realized that these places were the context of my life and somehow I must make them the subject matter of my art. I started to make drawings in meetings and used them as the basis of paintings. Rather than fleeing from the meetings, I deepened my involvement with them through art and brought them into my studio. While living in a natural environment next to the sea, I was making pictures of meetings.

I actually began to look forward to the meetings. I was as interested in the concept of transforming the sessions as I was in the pictures themselves. Other people in the meetings became intrigued, and I found that making the drawings helped me concentrate on business. The satisfaction that I received from the images must have been related to my intimate knowledge of the subject matter. I had empathy for bodily postures at conference tables and was familiar with the configurations of papers, water glasses, and coffee cups. I was painting the familiars of my work environment that previously had no connection to my art. It felt extraordinary to channel the feelings I had about office life into pictures. This existential milieu, a most unlikely subject matter for "art," began to generate what felt like an endless reservoir of intriguing and fresh images. I was able to engage all of my interests; everything came together. The artistic process helped me become more aesthetically attuned to offices, meetings, and daily life.

As I look back on those experiences, the meetings and the insulation project may have resulted in depression and stress because they were desanctified. Through art I was able to bring grace into my life. I took the things that were most bothersome and made them the subject matter of art. The toxin became the antitoxin, the medicine of art.

Relationships with other artists have been major influences on the formation of my therapeutic methods. I have sought out help from senior artists who have inspired and challenged me through their understanding of psyche and their innate therapeutic sensibilities. Rather than pursuing supervision with someone unfamiliar with the artistic process, I have continuously felt the need to activate the art therapy process within my private life through dialogue with artist mentors. Soul depends upon relationships with similar sensibilities in order to experience itself.

Vincent Ferrini is a master of the art/life interplay, and for the past twenty years we have had an unbroken dialogue about art's therapeutic properties. As he writes in *This Other Ocean, Books VI & VII of Know Fish*, his epic poem about contemporary life in Gloucester, Massachusetts, "I charge him . . . something is dancing between us . . . Psyche between us is enjoying the action of our theatre" (1991, p. 82).

In the studio of daily life we spontaneously enact an archetypal process of cooperative creating that is the basis of art as medicine. Socrates said his ideas "never come out of me; they always come from the person I am talking with." Nothing creates "in and by itself." When people and things interact, they are in a process of becoming "*for each other*" (Hamilton and Cairns, 1961, pp. 865–66).

Vincent's poem "Folksong" (1950/1976), which appeared in my 1981 book *The Arts and Psychotherapy*, has continued to embody the essential philosophy and method of my work in the arts and psychotherapy.

I pass
by day
   and night
no one has
   seen me

   If you ever
want to find
   me
and know me
   leave behind
yourself
   and enter
the caves
   of other
people

   there you
will find
   me
who is
   yourself

"Folksong" not only applies to relationships with people but guides my interactions with an image. Forgetting myself as best I can, I study the nature of the image, its colors, forms, and emotional qualities, and I open myself to its influences. This attitude is the basis of art as medicine. Imagination is the sympathetic medium in which dialoguing with images occurs, the faculty through which we establish compassion, understanding, and respect for things other than ourselves. Not only the world but our psyches are viewed as an ongoing interplay between varied figures and perspectives that emerge through creative action. Imaginative compassion for that which is other than myself is a constant artistic and ethical discipline.

Artistic images are not simply reflections of their makers and thus mirrors revealing the inner lives of artists. Richard Ellman, the author of literary biographies of James Joyce and Oscar Wilde, said that while it can be useful to clearly distinguish the creation from the artist, it is a "fallacy that the text is a virgin birth accomplished without human intervention" (1988, pp. 107–108). Our lives influence the nature of our paintings, dreams, stories, and other creations. As I say later in this book, images come through us like children, and they inherit biological and psychic traits. But like children, they have autonomous lives and souls that quickly begin to influence and change the lives of their makers.

Life does imitate art, as evidenced by how we change in response to images. We become what we imagine, as the person obsessed with troubling thoughts knows. It is the artistic imagination, and not the willful mind, that effortlessly transforms the torturing demon into an inspirational daimon. The discipline of changing an image or a story, rather than the moralistic commandment to change ourselves, eases the burden. As the images change, we change with them.

In Vincent Ferrini's play *Shadows Talking* (1991), a character says:

> If you could forget
> who you think you are
> you might catch up with
> what you really are
> & can't see—

Art is formed from life and passes back into it. This is the ecology of art as medicine, the *pas de deux* between art and life.

★   ★   ★

After experimenting with the transformation of conflict through art, my painting again attempted to align itself with the movements of the art therapy process. My art has always been responsive to patterns emerging from the therapeutic studio. I established an environment where people were able to paint from their souls, and their art in turn inspired my personal expression. The studio has always been ahead of me. I follow its lead. The purity and vitality of the soul art that people made in art therapy gave me a new standard to emulate. I wanted something that was indigenous to soul experience. I had devised an environment through which other people could contact archaic and primary processes of artistic expression, but I had not yet figured out how to do this for myself. The group environment of collaborative creation was inspirational, but I had not found a way to participate as a maker of images.

Art therapy's laudable emphasis on the well-being of patients and their art creates a dilemma for the art therapist's personal artistic expression. As we distance ourselves from our own inner expression, we increasingly lose an intimate personal relationship to the making of images.

The realization of the promise of art therapy calls for complete participation by art therapists. I have always believed that attending to others does not require me to stop expressing myself. It is often impossible for me to paint because of what I need to do for a person or a group, but there are also times when the studio benefits from my involvement as a co-creator. As I suggested earlier, using myself as an example, we art therapists often avoid painting because we fear self-revelation before our patients, clients, or students. Strict principles such as always refraining from personal expression sometimes function as a defense against co-involvement as an image maker. These tendencies are unconsciously influenced by the persistence of competitive values in contradiction to art therapy's stated belief that every image is significant. Art therapists are also inhibited in expressing themselves because they themselves become the subjects of the diagnostic perspective that dominates their work.

I have to keep reminding myself that it is the soul which ministers to itself through our art therapy studio. I am always liable to worry about how I will be perceived, forgetting that I am one of many aspects in soul's therapeutic studio and sometimes may contribute through a painting. The idea that we are all involved in soul's therapy liberates the art therapist from the dualistic relationship with clients. Without relinquishing roles and responsibilities, we are given another perspective on making art. The soul benefits from both therapists' and patients' involvement in expression.

My experience indicates that personal artistic expression by the art therapist furthers the creative energy of the studio. Working together with a group enables a different energy to appear than talking. Soul communicates with soul through the process of painting, and group members "sense" their leader in a different way. I have actually discovered that on days when I do not feel like painting, the group misses my involvement. It seems so important for art therapy to experiment with the complete range of its communications between therapists and participants and to avoid "absolute" role specifications, which generally evolve as modes of defense. If the soul of the therapist wants to paint, it is an expression of soul's purpose, and it will contribute to the therapeutic process. Groups support us in responding to these instincts when it is clear that our primary commitment is the well-being of the studio.

I have had to struggle with the ethics and purpose of self-expression during the therapeutic process because of the unstated taboo that art therapy has cast over the issue. Granted, I am primarily working in the retreat environment of residential group studios where the time structures are more liberal than the conventional therapeutic hour with a single patient. Yet I recall my work with the psychiatrist Robert Coles in the 1970s and his tendency to sit down and draw freely with the children he was interviewing, compare pictures, and generally help them feel more comfortable through his co-participation.

Music and dance therapists have always communicated with their clients through the languages of their art forms. The music therapist improvises together with the client and the dynamics of the music interaction, or lack of interaction, become the subject matter of the therapy. The process orientation of music therapy and the emphasis on musical communication and the transmission of its energies keep the relationship grounded in the medicine of the art.

Art therapists, by contrast, rarely communicate through their medium because their artistic values are not based on an interactive process, and this makes it unnatural for them to work together with clients. The object allows itself to be talked about in a way that is not possible with the moving expressions of music and dance. This quality has contributed to the tradition of diagnostic labeling that does not permeate the other creative arts therapies to the same degree. If images are generated by the patient for the purpose of diagnostic assessment, then it does lead to role confusion when the therapist paints.

When communicating with a patient through music, we are generally involved in a common and social art experience, as opposed to the solitary nature of painting. While making music with patients, my eyes and consciousness can observe their expression and attend to their needs. In a painting studio, personal involvement in my pictures makes it more challenging to watch what is going on around me. Before painting I will always drum for the group or silently watch and support them while they get started. When everyone is working freely, I may begin to work. I tend to combine painting with watching, moving about, and interacting with participants, encouraging them to visit me, and trying to be sensitive to the atmosphere of the group while painting. I have discovered that many participants will be positively influenced by this way of interacting and will adopt similar expressive styles in the group.

As I experimented with the role of co-painter within the studio, my pictures became increasingly influenced by themes and images that other people were painting. When I expressed old themes of my own, I felt as though I were defending myself from the influences of the studio and the challenge of engaging current images and feelings. Rather than fight against the appearance of "old themes" when I work in a studio, I now perceive them as familiars. As soon as I accept them, they change and adapt to the new context.

In our studios we experimented with the interpretation of images. As a leader I helped people to do things that I had not yet done myself. I watched graduate students and art therapy colleagues tell stories about paintings, talk with them, and make performances in response to the paintings with a depth and creativity that transformed my practice of art therapy.

When I began my work as a group therapist, I was consistently amazed at the way in which groups changed my feelings. If I entered a group depressed, I inevitably left in better spirits. The collective energy always affected me. The same thing happens to me in a painting studio. I am affected and inspired by the work of others. They stir the pot of creativity. It might be a specific painting that arouses my dormant expressive instincts, or it may be the simple fact that I am part of a group of people who are committed to painting. The one who convenes them for the sake of creative expression may also participate in the group's creative arousal. Again, the ethics of therapy have an unstated taboo against therapists using the therapeutic process to their personal advantage, but the dualistic values of clinical service establish an unnecessary confusion. We do not have to put into opposition the well-being of therapists and patients and insist on exclusive, one-way orientation that is against our ecological natures. Roles and responsibilities are certainly different, and these reflections on influences do not suggest relaxing moral vigilance. However, therapists should not feel reluctant or guilty to state that they personally benefit from therapeutic process.

Creative fulfillment for the art therapist as an artist will be recycled back into the work and service to others. I am an example of an art therapist who did not perceive his profession as a context for the creation of "serious" art. It took me years to realize that the art therapy studio is a vital stimulant for creation and an intelligent forum where I can show my work. Involved with the stereotypic notion of the solitary and "free" artist in his individual studio, I looked at my group work as a "job" where I put in my time helping others in order to someday achieve the ideal of working alone. I was so busy with what I did not have, and with my desire to live the stereotypical life of the artist, that I overlooked the riches of my immediate environment. The conventional ideal of the artist is tied to the desire for social acceptance. Ironically, it never occurred to me that the studio groups are little societies that can give individual painters the attention and inspiration that every artist needs. The members of these art therapy groups transformed my vision of art. They repeatedly demonstrate how every new group environment can become the nurturing, responsive, and affirming art world that every individual artist needs. The studios take art back to the intimate tribe with its shared rituals and beliefs. Fantasies of "recognition" by the world at large have grown from the impersonal and intangible patterns of mass culture.

Art as medicine implies a revisioning of values, and my experience suggests that consciousness has not caught up with what we are doing. The archetypal process of art therapy promises a revitalization of artistic expression that we have not yet assimilated.

Many artists view art as serious psychological inquiry: William Blake, D. H. Lawrence, Frida Kahlo, Charlotte Salomon, the surrealists. Art therapy can contribute to this tradition by furthering art's potential as depth psychology. Pioneering depth psychologists such as C. G. Jung and Otto Rank realized that the arts are the channels through which the soul speaks, but the early twentieth century was heavily biased toward a scientific perspective on psyche. Although methods of inquiry and expression were based on the use of images, therapy and psychology were viewed as science rather than art. "Men of science," rather than artists, were the authorities on the psychological significance of art because it was assumed that psyche's speech had to be translated into clinical language in order to be understood.

As an art therapist, my mission has not been in opposition to science. However, I have been committed to liberating art and art therapy from the narrow perspectives of scientism which have discouraged artists from realizing their potential as psychological savants. It is time to acknowledge the interplay between art, psychology, and psychotherapy as one of this century's contributions to the work of the soul. My vision of art therapy builds on this history.

A Link to the "Art World"

> The blessings experienced in therapy can reach further: they can remind artists everywhere what the function of art has always been and will always be.
>
> —RUDOLF ARNHEIM (1992)

THE EMINENT MUSEUM director Sherman Lee once said, "Our first responsibility is to the object, and to the person who wants to respond to it in a private way. Art is not therapy . . . or social uplift, and a museum is not a community center" (Temin, 1991).

Although Sherman Lee is committed to the worthy goal of furthering the integrity and artistic standards of museums, his comments reveal the poorly informed and pervasive sentiment in the art community *against* art therapy. The dismissal of the social and therapeutic "aspects" of art can be an unnecessary defense against contamination by mass culture. Art therapy and revolutionary art can be practiced in ways that maintain the highest ideals of art history. If art therapy is to align itself with the history of art, it must demonstrate a sincere and intelligent treatment of the object together with a commitment to the making of significant art works. The protectors of art have to witness our sense of responsibility "to the object, and to the person who wants to respond to it in a private way." Ironically, Lee's statement against art therapy articulates my vision of what it is.

Surrealism may be art therapy's clearest link to twentieth-century art. During the surrealist era many of the values that currently guide art as medicine began to take shape. Surrealism, like art therapy, is a philosophy and method of fully engaging art with life and psyche. Art becomes a ritual act that opens people to the experience of soul. The art object is a psychic tool rather than a commercial commodity, and the aesthetic contemplation of paintings is encouraged as a way to experience "surreality." André Breton described surrealism as "based on a belief in the superior reality of certain forms of previously neglected associations, in the omnipotence of the dream, in the disinterested play of thought. . . . I believe in the future resolution of these two states, dream and reality, which are seemingly so contradictory, into a kind of absolute reality, a *surreality*" (1969, pp. 26, 14).

Although Breton advocated an aesthetic "disinterest," he nevertheless presents surreality as a higher reality and catches himself in the trap of reason's judgments. This undermines his goal of calling our attention to the reality of imagination, a reality free from comparative judgments. But surrealism's immersion in the grist of urban daily life and its systematic efforts to achieve social transformation anticipate art as medicine.

Surrealism embraced the art of "the insane" and celebrated its "total authenticity" as a standard for the renewal of art itself. Breton felt that art criticism creates "a suffocating smokescreen of incense . . . around a few consecrated artists," and because of this bias the standard of art never "strays from the miserable little guideline they have drawn" (1972, p. 315). He celebrated Frida Kahlo's art as "a ribbon around a bomb . . . pure surreality" (ibid., p. 144) and was delighted that her work was conceived without knowledge of the surrealist movement.

In art therapy we also speak of "authenticity" as the principal determinant of quality. Soul painting emerges as a universal genre that embodies what Prinzhorn described as fundamental "psychic forms of expression."

In addition to its commitment to emotional authenticity and social activism, surrealism's correspondence with art therapy includes universal participation, methods of automatic expression, the importance of dreams, and the creation of art works that involve a dynamic interplay between artist and audience.

Breton's revolt was focused on art's exclusivity. He took delight in vital expressions outside the anointed sphere. The professional discipline of art history tends to deal with a circumscribed and closed group of artists rather than with the complete phenomenon of art. Feminist scholars are demonstrating that many stories have not been told. Women and men who are not part of the designated chain of influences that art historians follow are forgotten, and may never have been recognized in the first place.

When we focus exclusively on the linear history of personalities and movements, we overlook the deeper and more mysterious archetypal art history of images and creative processes. By limiting art history to the way in which a select group of people influence one another, the industry of art establishes an aristocratic bloodline of artists. Whatever these quasi-divinities touch is transformed into treasure. The rest of us can come onto the scene only as "outsider artists." Those who do not "make it" while they are alive hope that the angels of fame will come posthumously, as in the case of Vincent Van Gogh.

If we look at art history from an archetypal perspective, we will concentrate on images and psychic processes, not just lineage. For example, within the archetypal context the orderly mind of historical classification freely interacts with its labyrinthian shadow; memory jostles with forgetting; progress is tempered by interruption. Change, recurrence, and other forces are personified, with humans serving as their instruments of expression. Purpose takes the form of a dialogue between characters, an exchange that does not fit exclusively into a progressive pattern. Every time a singular, exclusive, or absolute view is presented, its shadows are unconsciously activated. Nothing is fixed, yet the archetypal movements are eternal. Within this context art history becomes a pantheon of varied forces, or images, and human beings function as their agents.

The interaction between what we see and what we do not see takes on new relevance, and history is imagined as a record of stories untold. As Yeats said of reality, "From nowhere into nowhere nothing's run."

We can also reverse the poet's statement and say, "From everywhere into everywhere everything runs." History, of the archetypal sort, is a process in which stories of infinite variety are constantly being told.

Psychic automatism was the dominant feature of surrealist aesthetics. It was based on a belief that psyche's movements are not only purposeful but wondrous, and that the reasoning mind can limit our perceptions of reality. The dream was considered to be psyche's most splendid form of automatic expression, and therefore surrealist art came as close as possible to the pure dream experience. The world of the dream became the basis of a new interpretation of art, engaging all people. Since pure surrealism advocated a "total spontaneity of expression" as experienced in dreams, the *trompe-l'oeil* representation of dream images of Dali and others was regarded as a "still-life deception" by Breton. They are conceptual and technical as contrasted to Breton's vision—more fixed than fluid. Although William Rubin referred to the literal painting of dream images by Magritte, Tanguy, and Dali as "academic illusionism," he described how these painters and their more spontaneous counterparts, Miró and Masson, were all involved with "poetic painting": "The common denominator of all this painting was a commitment to subjects of a visionary, poetic, and hence metaphoric order, thus the collective appellation, *peinture-poésie*, or poetic painting" (1968, p. 64).

The similarity of subject matter in art therapy and in surrealism emerges from common interests in what I call "imaginal realism." Automatism advocated more than "depicting" psychic experiences that had already taken place. Rather than literally painting a particular memory of a dream image, the automatic strain of surrealism advocated painting from a dreamlike state. Desiring a more direct engagement of inner movements, the artist's painting process and style corresponded to the movements of psyche. Breton described how automatism "gave *wings* to the artist's hand."

> Not content simply to trace the shape of objects, this hand, enamoured of its own movement and of that alone, described the involuntary figures within which, as experience has shown, these shapes were destined to become re-embodied. Indeed, the essential discovery of surrealism is that, without preconceived intention, the pen that flows in order to write and the pencil that runs in order to draw *spin* an infinitely precious substance which, even if not always possessing an exchange value, none the less appears charged with all the emotional intensity stored up within the poet or painter at a given moment. (1972, p. 68)

Psyche's images emerged through the hand, which acts as an intermediary between the materials and the consciousness of the painter. The hand is truly "between" different worlds and therefore cannot be completely tied to either one. The surrealists used religious terms, "emanations" and "manifestations," to describe the images that appeared through their spontaneous movements, but it would be misleading to suggest that the entire painting process from beginning to end was automatic. In art therapy, automatic gestures help to get pictures started and are useful when a person is blocked. Automatism is a mode of emanation, often liberating and invigorating, which provides access to unexpected and fresh subject matter. Images emerge and carry the energy of the initial expressive gestures. Artists have found automatism to be a mode of "redemption," both in terms of their work as a whole and as a means of resolving individual pictures. However, there is a complementary process of shaping, changing, and reflecting upon spontaneous manifestations that characterizes the work of even the most radical automatists.

Psychic automatism influenced all of the great art and psychology of the early twentieth century—Joyce, Proust, Freud, Jung, and others like D. H. Lawrence, who valued creations that "come unwatched out of one's pen." Since this trend cannot be reduced to a single source, automatism fits into our notion of archetypal art history. It is an ongoing and distinct movement that manifests itself through many different individuals.

Nietzsche was a significant influence through the content of his thought and through his spontaneous methods of expression. His belief that consciousness was a deterrent to the "creative-affirmative" force of instinct seems to be the bedrock of everything related to psychic automatism. Prinzhorn's vitalism, rooted in the tradition of Nietzsche, suggests that the creative instinct is present in every person together with other primal traits. In his first book, *The Birth of Tragedy*, Nietzsche introduced the idea of art as medicine: "Here, when the danger to his will is greatest, *art* approaches as a saving sorceress, expert at healing. She alone knows how to turn these nauseous thoughts about the horror or absurdity of existence into notions with which one can live" (1967, p. 60).

Freud's use of free association closely paralleled surrealist methods of automatism, but his scientism was not compatible with their interest in furthering mystery. While Freud used expressions of the psyche as material for a new science, for the surrealists they were revelations and objects of wonder, *le merveilleux* (the marvelous). Surrealism's concern for ordinary things and the place of art in daily life leads to art as medicine. The painter René Magritte saw surrealism as a liberation from artistic censors that people inherit and that obstruct appreciation of the marvelous in everyday experience.

Automatism is as fundamental to art therapy as it is to surrealism. We have become accustomed to artists and therapists saying, "Trust the process. Relax and follow its lead. Let it speak through you. Don't try to control it. Open to that which appears from outside your frame of reference."

The early explorations of art in psychoanalysis often focused on forming images from preliminary scribbles. Automatic forms of expression are essential to my art therapy studios, where we help people to paint kinetically, from the body, in order to avoid the stifling restrictions of the mind that tells the hand what it "should" paint. Mind-based images are typically stiff forms, painted primarily through the hand and wrist, and they do not engage the full resources of the body. Rather than restricting ourselves to automatic scribbles coordinated by the hand and eye, we encourage kinetic painting that enlists elements of dance. People imagine themselves dancing when they begin to paint, using both hands and arms as well as the body as a whole. Movement generates vital and instinctual images that avoid the restrictions of mental planning.

Within the surrealist revolution, the dream not only served as the model of automatic expression and psychic emanation but also affirmed the ability of every person to generate unusual imagery. According to the surrealist ideal, "art would be a *means* of expression, an instrument of self-discovery, not an *end* to be savored" (Rubin, 1968, p. 64). This goal was never achieved within the "art world," where surrealist paintings were bought, sold, and conserved as objects of great value. Art therapy, however, has succeeded in fulfilling surrealism's revolutionary aesthetic of expression for its own sake. In spite of its rhetoric, surrealism always savored and appreciated images, *le merveilleux*, as charms and stimulants activating further expression.

The attitudes and methods of painters in the therapeutic studio are not significantly different from what one experiences when working in isolation or in an art school. In both situations manifestations of psychic life may be experienced in the painting process and images. The differences between therapeutic and academic perspectives are largely determined by how people "treat" art objects and one another. Surrealism laid the groundwork for art as medicine, allowing the witness of a work of art to become an active participant, a part of the life of an image as it exists in a particular moment. The surrealists perceived the art object as a psychic functionary, operating within an environment that was also a mode of transformation.

Surrealist values were antithetical to images as private treasures and commodities. However, the painters involved in the surrealist movement were also part of the gallery traditions of Western art, which used surrealism to further their commercial aims and to generate yet another category of commodity. Further, surrealist painters responded to the historical context of the gallery art that preceded them, and they had a significant influence on the next generation of artists. Their rebellion actually advanced the system they were opposing. The only way to make the revolutionary vision a practical reality was to establish a new context and a new aesthetic perspective to which the artist is totally committed. Art therapy may have realized this surrealist ambition.

Surrealism was handicapped by its inability to separate itself from the heroic ideal of the artist, an ideal which reinforced the economics of establishing the value of an art object according to the individual's reputation. Although automatism tried to imagine art as expressing archetypal psyche as well as the individual, a supportive context for this transformation did not yet exist. Art therapy has achieved this goal largely because it was never part of either the market or the heroic tradition and therefore it has nothing to lose by disregarding them. Serious and gifted artists who long for a creative life of soul-making are being drawn into art therapy. Our work is taking place with great vitality and in full correspondence with art's archetypal processes of healing and psychic expression.

We have received considerable inspiration from the surrealist commitment to an immediate art experience or event that cannot occur without witnesses. There was a sacramental quality to surrealism, making the arts a means through which le merveilleux was experienced by gatherings of people. The sacrament is a sensible sign for the invisible, the divine, and the arts are twentieth-century vehicles for the celebration of what André Breton, who was nicknamed "the pope," called the "modern mystery." The word surreality itself was a restatement and revitalization of the divine.

Surrealism called for the participation of the entire society in the dissolution of separations between art and life. Their criticisms of art focused on the social context and its values. To them, everyone had equal access to creation, and the artist became an exemplary or shamanic figure who enacted the "holy madness" of the community.

Artists fashioned themselves into works of art, following Nietzsche, who said fifty years earlier: "He is no longer an artist, he has become a work of art" (1967, p. 37). What really mattered was the impersonal and spontaneous process of creation, which transforms everything, including the artists themselves.

I am convinced that, like Nietzsche, the surrealists wanted to use a sacred sense of shamanic ecstasy and enchantment as a means of revitalizing the world. These artists were closer to the archetype of the shaman than to that of the mythic hero. If they sought to become "semidivinities," they also desired to use themselves as intermediaries for the resanctification of life. They were reenacting the shamanic archetype of reviving the *anima mundi*. Their sacred values offered alternatives to art as an economic industry. In *The Breasts of Tiresias* Apollinaire (1956) describes how the dramatist becomes "God the Creator" within the universe of the play, which doesn't "photograph" life but "brings forth" life.

Apollinaire is speaking poetically and is not literally suggesting that humans replace divinities but rather that divine or daimonic life flows through us in a process that we understand as creativity. Every person has the ability to be an agency of this force. Through involvement in the creative process we bring forth life, fashioning it, and ourselves, anew.

By making themselves the "objects" of art, the surrealists strove to demystify the heroic artist. The creator became an "object" who was himself reshaped by the artistic process. They attacked egotism and rational humanism, anticipating Hillman's belief (echoing Jung) that the psyche is not in us—we are in the psyche (1977b, p. 173). We humans are part of art's subject matter.

By shifting the position of the artist from subject to object, Dada and surrealism anticipate art's therapeutic role. The reasoning mind, rather than being the controlling instrument of therapy, is one of many things that is acted upon by art's medicine. In keeping with the ancient Hellenic cult of Asklepios, the ego incubates or actually goes to sleep so that it can be acted upon by external remedies. While one sleeps in the house of Asklepios, "the god is expected to give instructions in a dream or else to effect a direct cure" (Burkert, 1985, p. 215).

Creative energy acts upon us, so that the artist, as object, is changed by the process. But artists as patients are not entirely passive. They do initiate the process by preparing the context and the materials (including themselves), opening to the movements of creation and learning how to shape its emanations.

As shamanic figures, the surrealist artists used their creativity to help others to participate in "surreality." Like the shaman they took risks and used surprise, shock, and dramatic provocations to establish bonds with others. Their primary objective was the creation of a *temenos* where all could become immersed in a shared surreality. In art therapy I have rarely encountered a group that was not capable of giving an intelligent and compassionate response to art. The audience has to be prepared for the event, however, and must fully accept its validity. If the audience is confused about the purpose of the event, if they are distrustful or uneasy, or if they have doubts about the relevance of the process, then the experience will not evoke the sense of safety and support that opens the heart and soul. The surrealists, like the shaman and the creative arts therapist, staged art experiences before audiences that understood and participated in their sacramental dimension.

This aspect of surrealism anticipated the role of the therapist as a witness and guide who participates in a shared art experience with others. The paintings and the persons are transformed through forces evoked by the audience and the surrounding environment. People present themselves and their work in order to experience the transformative effects of a *rite de passage*. A person might present a simple stone or household artifact that initially arouses little interest. But as the objects are used in performances, or after the owner tells a story about how they embody significant events and passages, they are "ensouled" and alive for everyone in the group. The objects are animated by the attention they receive.

People looking at the object do not "give" soul to it. They witness and affirm the soul qualities that are already present but unseen. The same applies to persons. The group affirms the life of the soul that is active in all of us but which goes unseen and unacknowledged.

The engagement of soul occurs when people speak directly to one another about what they are experiencing. I was in a group recently where an art therapist responded to a woman's art by saying, "If I look at your picture as a clinician, I will ask why you put that face off to the side of the picture." The statement assumes that there is a psychological reason for the composition, that the artist is responsible for the face's placement, and that its location refers to something in the artist's psyche. If the artist replied by saying, "I don't know why I put it there," the "clinical" mindset assumes that she is avoiding disclosure.

Perhaps the face wanted to be off to the side of the picture. It may have put itself there. Or the artist's hand, acting independently from the mind, put it there. Some things are not to be explained by the artist's motivations.

I have always been irritated by egocentric assumptions that the image fits into the *a priori* theoretical bias of the interpreter. The woman who made the face was herself intrigued by its placement. She was not denying its unusual nature. She was open to talking about how she responded to its qualities, and she was eager to hear how other people experienced the image. If the art therapist had stepped out of the authoritative role of expert clinician and asked the face in the painting why it placed itself off to the side of the picture, there would have been a different quality to the question. It would have evoked imagination rather than explanation.

In art therapy we see how the environment of the studio is transformed when people begin to interact creatively with their pictures. When this shift occurs, the feeling tone immediately changes, imagination enters the room, and an unconscious sense of sacred spectacle, safety, and support from others is established.

In a foreword that Helen Landgarten asked me to write for her most recent book (1991), I said that many of us involved with art therapy are "refugees and immigrants" from art's elitist and self-serving values, which have not provided access to the depths of the psyche "since the revolutionary days of the surrealists." Art therapy, like surrealism, focuses on using the creative process to treat and attend to the other, thriving on collaborations with other disciplines. Art as medicine reveals how the interaction of painting and psychotherapy deepens both. Landgarten's book emphasizes that art therapy is synergistic with virtually any theory or method of therapy. To me this suggests that the significance of images will never be exhausted by either theories *or* markets. The commercial art world is allied with a particular set of economic values, and we make an error when we perceive this context to be the exclusive or the highest realm of art.

For those of us in art therapy who desire to participate as full citizens in the community of art and its history, the revival of surrealist principles may offer access. If we want art history's attention, we have to speak its language and acknowledge its traditions. Art as medicine, like surrealism, is a manifestation of art's desire to connect psyche, the dream, the suffering soul, and the daily lives of other people.

Psyche's Movement

The universe really is motion and nothing else.
—SOCRATES

IN OUR "POSTMODERN" era of therapy there is a realization that ancient notions of illness as spirit possession have their merits, providing alternatives to the sometimes impossible pressures to change the self.

Socrates chastised the physicians of his day for attempting to heal the body without first engaging the soul. "You must begin" he said to Charmides, "by curing the soul—that is the first and essential thing." Soul is closer to process—ongoing movement—than it is to fixity. Medicines that treat the soul must therefore have a kinetic nature. In Plato's *Dialogues* Socrates spoke to Theaetetus about how everything is generated from "a flowing stream of change" that "keeps things fresh": "All the things we are pleased to say 'are,' really are in process of becoming, as a result of movement and change and of blending one with another. We are wrong to speak of them as 'being,' for none of them ever is; they are always becoming" (Hamilton and Cairns, 1961, p. 857).

I imagine soul as *kinesis*, process, creation, interplay, and continuous motion. *Soul* is generally synonymous with *psyche*, but it suggests particular and individualized conditions. It is a word that philosophers and artists have always used to suggest the essential vitality of a person, thing, or the world itself. Loss of soul is a "stuck" condition in which the flow has stopped. Psychology speaks of "fixations" as defenses against change. The "fixed" idea is nonvolatile, stationary. Artists accustomed to a vital kinesis of imagination fear the prospect of "drying up." The soulless state is one of desiccation, when "the currents" no longer run.

A woman in an art therapy retreat painted a series of expressionist paintings in which the flow and movement of paint, forms, colors, and texture were more apparent than the presence of figures. The pictures were energetic and beautifully crafted. When the artist commented upon the images, she focused on figures (trees, flying persons, children, animals, monsters) that other people in the group did not see. The stories that she told about her pictures expressed a longing for professional fulfillment and her difficulty in accepting her life as it is. She spoke of how this pattern of looking for what she does not have makes it difficult to see her paintings and feel the presence of soul.

The rest of us saw how the paintings were bursting with energy. We suggested that she was already where she wanted to be, but she could not see or feel it. She chose to concentrate on the partially hidden figures when talking about her pictures and overlooked the vital bio-energetics of the work as a whole. She was thinking in terms of fixed forms rather than pictorial movement.

When we are "stuck" in our imagework, we typically have left the image and become enveloped in thoughts. Change can result by simply looking carefully at the physical qualities of the picture and taking a different perspective on its relationship to our life. We call this move restating or reframing.

I do not want to give the impression that we are always replacing negative stories with positive ones. Often the process may lead to just the opposite. Through restatement we shift perspectives and see that "stuckness" comes from rigidly following what Blake called "single vision."

"Stuckness" is an absence of movement and the inability to perceive motion in the moment.

Motion has its pathological aspects in manic flights or perseverative rigidities. Art as medicine stays on course as long as we "stick with the image," as recommended by Rafael López-Pedraza. This simple maxim of archetypal psychology is the soul guide of the work. It means staying with the medium, the process, and the artistic discipline, whether it be drama, movement, poetry, music, or painting. "Sticking with the image" includes staying with sounds, gestures, body movements, feelings, environments, and other aspects of art forms. When we leave the image, we leave the context and the presence of soul. Our method is sustained communion with "the other," the image or painting. "Sticking with images" is not static and distinctly different from being "stuck." Our "sticking" is kinetic, a flexible movement with images. Soul moves through our interaction with paint. Aristotle's peripatetic style of teaching corresponded to the movements that his philosophy expressed. He was immersed in the imagination of motion. The same can be said about our view of the act of painting and the accompanying interpretive meditations.

Staying with the image demonstrates how the object before us is an opening to soul. We find "depth" on the surface of the image, in the details of its presentation. In my art therapy studios we not only stay in contact with the image but we "go with it" through its transformations and movements. This is a movement therapy where we travel together, accompany one another, become familiars, and witness changes. When people open to art's suggestions, they change as they watch images change.

The shamanic definition of illness as soul loss corresponds to the lost soul as a lost image, a lost presence. Whenever two or more people working with a painting find themselves involved in tangential conversations during which they lose contact with one another as well as with their feelings, returning to the specific qualities of a painting will restore a deeper, more immediate sense of relationship. The other person helps me to concentrate on the presence of the image, which, as mutual object of concentration, becomes a link between us. Intensifying my focus on the image actually helps to deepen my relationship with the other person. We become involved in a sort of ritual that transcends our individual reflections. The image and the particulars of the environment are conduits for the experience of soul. "Sticking with the image" is a restatement of the Gnostic passage "Recognize what is before your eyes, and what is hidden will be revealed to you" (the Gospel of Thomas).

The process of staying with images applies to every aspect of the art therapy experience, from the first phases of making a painting to the dialogues we have with it afterward. The most effective way to work with people suffering from acute psychosis is to help them make perceptual contact with images in a therapy of attunement to the structural features of the environment. "Can you see red in the picture? Can you touch it? Where is the doorway? How many trees are in the picture on the left? Which color attracts your eye first?" These simple questions evoke a sense of presence. Feelings of attunement to environments and movements are the basis of our therapy.

My early use of art in treating psychosis concentrated on just this phenomenological process of becoming aware of what was present in the image (McNiff, 1973, 1974). We always began by looking at the physical qualities of pictures, and discovered that everyone in a group, therapists and patients alike, has a limited awareness during preliminary observations of paintings. Through a sustained process of viewing and discussing pictures, our perceptions became more differentiated and visually aware.

Preliminary observations are typically carried out through habitual modes of perception that do not give us time to be affected by the image and changed by it. Looking at the image becomes a meditation. The longer we look, the more we see, and the more the image influences consciousness.

Staying with the image is as essential to the psychological interpretation of paintings as it is to the structural analysis that I have just described. The depth and precision of psychological reflection is determined by the extent to which it corresponds to the physical characteristics of the image. The two modes of inquiry are closely connected.

In my work, the psychological dialogue is always based upon a careful observation of the structural aspects of the image. The feelings we have about the image, the stories we tell about how we made it, the reminiscences it evokes, the things that the images say to us, and the things that we say to them are always closely attuned to physical qualities. We focus on the visual qualities of the specific tree, animal, color, or shape rather than speak about them in a generalized way. I am more interested in a careful observation of the details of the particular tree that is drawn than a general discussion about the significance of "trees." Psychological significance comes from relating these visual characteristics to the intimate details of the interpreter's life.

We view interpretations as metaphors, verbal responses to the image, analogies that we make to other aspects of our lives, and translations of the visual image into other art forms—poetry, movement, sound, performance. Art is constantly being interpreted by art in a sequential process of creation, metaphoric movement, and image-making that refreshes the soul. Our medicine views interpretation as an unending process of attunement.

Some might take "sticking with the image" as an interpretive fundamentalism that discourages responses not structurally present in the image. The maxim is not intended as an authoritarian doctrine of literal observation. And I do not think it inhibits the imaginative transformations of art. The method is intended to affirm the presence of "the other" and to assure that our creative responses do not deviate from treating the actual image before us.

Painters are likely to have more than one response to their pictures, and this multiplicity affirms the generative powers of art. It also manifests the variability of human tastes and observations. The singular presence of the physical image prevents the variety of responses from becoming chaotic or fragmenting. Our meditations are always grounded in the presence of a particular picture.

Responses that stay close to the actual structure and qualities of the painting are likely to stimulate feelings of connectedness among the people involved, a condition that I have described as evoking a sense of soulfulness. The Latin origins of the word *religion* derive from the "binding together" of elements, which was applied to "bonds" between humans and gods. When someone in art therapy loses contact with the specific painting while speaking about it, there is a sense that the soul connection is severed. It is regained by reconnecting with the object of contemplation.

By focusing on "binding together," the complementary perspective of "letting go" is activated. The bonds of staying with the image are flexible and never permanent. I must let go of the painting with which I was just involved in order to engage the one before me. There is an instinctual rhythm and timing in the process as in our biological functions and social interactions. In order to do this work with images, we train our sensitivities to open to what presents itself, and this cannot be done unless we let go of the prior involvement.

Simone Weil described how unusual it is to find a person who can truly listen to another. She said: "The soul empties itself of all of its contents in order to receive into itself the being it is looking at, just as he is, in all his truth" (quoted in Hellman, 1984, p. 87). We "let go" of thoughts in order to truly witness. The process is a continuous motion of coming together and letting go, guided by the spirit of mutual sensitivity. Confusion enters when we lose contact with the image, with one another, with breath, and when we are taken over by spirits of panic and distrust.

When we stay with the image that presents itself within a particular context, the image gathers people together around a common focus. It does the same for all of "the participants" within ourselves, the many different voices and figures who are for the moment fused into a shared commitment. This is the eternal function of ritual and meditation—to bring a focus on something "other."

Jane Harrison's reflections on ritual suggest that the process of staying open to the "other" is an ongoing meditation:

> The only intelligible meaning that ritual has for me, is the keeping open of the individual soul—that bit of the general life which life itself has fenced in by a separate organism—to other souls, other separate lives, and to the apprehension of other forms of life. The avenues are never closed. Life itself, physical and spiritual, is the keeping of them open. Whether any systematized attempt to remind man, by ritual, of that whole of life of which he is a specialized fragment can be made fruitful or not, I am uncertain. (1962, p. 553)

We are always changing, and consciousness is forever challenged to become aware of where we are. The "stuck" consciousness clings to obsessions and repeated stories and does not open to new terrain. There is a reluctance to take a risk, and it protects itself from the realignments and demands that changes make in the daily structure of our lives. The "new" is an expression of "renewal," or what Harrison describes as "keeping open," an archetypal process that responds to the soul's need for movement and fresh engagements.

In the art therapy profession there are long-standing separations between process and product, art *as* therapy and art *in* therapy, and so forth. A graduate student from a midwestern university once telephoned me for an interview with a standard list of questions generated by her seminar: "Are you process- or product-oriented in your practice of art therapy? Do you believe in art *as* therapy or art *in* therapy? What is your theoretical orientation: psychoanalytic, humanistic, developmental, behavioral?"

I answered her questions by examining the dualistic, either-or perspectives in which they were framed, and as a result we had an animated conversation that probably did reveal my "theoretical bias." The questions, in keeping with behavioral science data-gathering, assume that the person is in one box or the other. They are based upon fixed classifications, in contrast to an interplay that allows the perspectives to collaborate. Every situation is a convergence. Art is therapeutic, and therapy makes use of art. Psyche is a pantheon populated by varied points of view, none of which is free of contradictions.

If we allow this sense of interplay, we do not have to oppose process to product. Paintings can indeed be seen as finished objects that emerge from the creative process, but this view overlooks the protean aspect of paintings, the building up and breaking down, the covering, the shifts, transformations, changes, and interrelations that comprise the psychophysics of constructing images from paint. The traditional view of painting sees only the last phase of the action, and as a result not enough attention is given to watching the image in its changing forms and presentations. We miss the movement. The *process* of painting reveals the working of metempsychosis, where there is a transmigration of soul from one phase of the product to another. These are the partners *with whom we move* while painting. The interpretation of images is also a sequence of acts, requiring sensitivity to movement. Rather than fixing meanings to images, we see them as participants in the soul's dance and what Paul Valéry called "total movement."

Artists who think too much about "final" products distance themselves from the product in front of them. Their thoughts reach beyond the manifestation at that particular phase. Like dreams, art works are surprising syntheses of elements on the threshold of consciousness that *present themselves*. The artist prepares the space and lets the controlling mind step aside. Artistic cognition responds and takes advantage of accidents, chance, lines, forms, figures, and interactions that emerge "unwatched." The responsive skill shapes these visitations into the style of the artist, which is continuously renewed through the interplay.

The intense desire to "break through" to the core of creativity is often itself the cause of "paralysis," yet another condition of arrested movement. Within this state, expression is characteristically tight, stiff, forced, and overworked rather than fluid, effortless, and graceful. Attention to the rhythms of breath and simple movements helps to restore a vital process that makes use of whatever presents itself during the day. Dreams teach us how this is done. Ordinary things bring us to what is alive and moving in the immediate context. Homer's *Odyssey* describes how "the soul flies out" of things "to hover like a dream."

The sources of imagination hover in the commonplace. Excessive thoughts about what I should be painting interfere with the ability to see what I am doing. Heroic expectations are blindfolds, obstructing the spontaneous response to what arrives independently of my intent.

Art's medicine, like that of the dream, involves the unexpected as a predictable expression of psyche's movement.

Emphasis on the reflexive aspects of artistic thought does not negate the inspirational importance of "visions" and ideals. The visions of artists function as activators of expression, while actual execution of the creative process is closer to the responsive sensitivity that I have described. Once the movement begins, I must respond to the leads that present themselves in the situation. If I remain fixed on an idea, I lose contact with immediate opportunities.

Memories also contribute to the interplay, but they must accommodate themselves to the present situation. Images from our personal treasuries of experience slip in and out of consciousness and fuel creation. I have never referred to this positive function as "the unconscious." In addition to abrogating the psychic aspects of memory, the idea of the unconscious replaces the richer, more evocative and positive image of soul. I use the word *unconscious* as a reference to that of which I am not aware, as a quality of consciousness or of its absence.

Viewing art as an expression of "the unconscious" assumes that consciousness is limited to reasoning. This attitude devalues the intelligence of the senses, the "thought of the heart," the thinking hand and eye, and the thoughtfulness of the moving body. Analysis is an esteemed participant in the making of art, but it is not the director of the operation. It is only one of the many facets of the psyche. Art as medicine enables therapy to use these varied faculties. Its principle contribution is the ability to reframe the entire opus of therapy. Rather than logically analyzing symptoms and reducing them to a rational sequence of causes, the artistic process may instead transform the scenario, completely restate the story and begin again, or replace the obsession with aesthetic contemplation. Many of our psychic maladies are in fact caused by the overactive mind, and exclusively analytic therapies may deepen the quagmire.

Art assuages through attunement to soul's movements and subtle vibrations. Rhythmic music, dance, poetry, and painting affirm a soul-state that exists independently of the individual human being. When I am drumming with a group of people, we move toward a common rhythm that contains us all. The drummer, dancer, and painter make contact with an *a priori* rhythm that guides and drives their expression. Rhythm and soul are to the artist what wind and water are to the sailor. They are forces with which the human creator interacts. They are not faculties that we possess. The soul generates images in cooperation with the artist.

Beginning artists, seasoned professionals, and anxious adults who have not touched paint since childhood all need help in learning how to become agencies of sincere expression. Artists with radically different degrees of technical expertise are afflicted by an inability to value the image for what it is. The acceptance of the significance of every gesture made, every color applied, and every feeling generated by the image establishes the context for psychological reflection and dialogue. This orientation does not deny the desire of the painter to "get it right"; to shape the image as well as possible; to change and transform colors, textures, and figures; to return to paintings at later dates and "fix" them; to take pleasure in the refinement of craft and sensitivity; et cetera. I can learn how to make a painting more aggressive, more provocative, more pastoral, more atmospheric, and so forth.

Technique is vitally important to art therapy. But we can begin only where we find ourselves at any given time. Whatever we do at that moment is the opening to soul. The errors, frustrations, changes, and desires to shape the image as well as possible are the contents of the psychological dialogue. They are the current figures of the painter's imagination.

Engaging conflicts of the moment fuels art: desire is paired with receptivity to whatever arrives; ambition is tempered by a delight in what I am doing at the present time; technical skills are furthered by constant experimentation with new possibilities rather than perfunctory implementation; the need to change may be a defense against the depth of the moment; the adoration of the present can protect me from the terrors and upheavals of change; ecstatic and automatic flights of expression are examined by the dispassionate eye of aesthetic judgment; what is considered to be noble obscures the splendor of what is seen as debased; everything is in motion, and all of the factors influence one another in collaborative pairs.

Destruction, the shadow of technical proficiency, is essential to creation. The creator is paired with a destructive power that serves as a companion and collaborator rather than as an adversary. Once the process is initiated, it is to be trusted. Destruction is a prelude to reconstruction.

Terry Netter, one of my painting professors in college, wrote to me that he is intrigued by the idea of art therapy because his art has always torn him apart. Reflecting upon the role of destruction in the creative process, it seems my sense of myself may have to dissolve in order for me to experience that which is not myself. If I resist and oppose this creative dissolution, it might have to increase its pressure. Shamanic initiation universally involves visions of psychic death and seeing one's skeleton. Theodore Roethke's poem "In a Dark Time" affirms that the soul's seeing may require a dark light.

Birkin in D. H. Lawrence's *Women in Love* describes how the mind must immerse itself in darkness, "everything must go," in order to experience transformation into another state of being:

> In our night-time, there's always the electricity switched on, we watch ourselves, we get it all in the head, really. You've got to lapse out before you can know what sensual reality is, lapse into unknowingness, and give up your volition. You've got to do it. You've got to learn not-to-be, before you can come into being. (1950, p. 48)

As creative arts therapists we are often so involved with making sure people have a "good" and "pleasant" experience with art that we do not see that soul might prefer "tearing apart" these positive intentions. It might need chaos rather than order, depression rather than happiness, ugliness rather than beauty, destruction rather than creation, and aggression rather than tranquillity. Therapists who try to impose "good feelings" on expressions bent on outrage will find themselves the target of the revolution.

Our therapies have been so intent upon strengthening egos that we have overlooked the medicine of what Keats called "self-destroying." Rather than belittle the ego and its contributions, we hope to regenerate its expressive partners and collaborators. Also, the destructuring aspects of creation are not always aggressive. Shifts in perspective can involve a gentle process of letting go. This strong medicine of destruction is not to be taken literally as the "self-destroying" of a person's life. Lawrence and Keats refer to the destructive "aspect" of creation, the breaking down that accompanies construction.

Images are our co-participants in creative activity. There is an intimate relationship between artists and their paintings but instead of seeing images as graphic signs of the artist's inner nature, we can imagine them as children, psychic offspring. They issue from us but lead autonomous lives. We nourish the images, profoundly determine their configurations, and shape them in our styles, but they will never be mirror reflections of us. Although the pictures we make are influenced by the contextual scenes of our lives, our different interests, obsessions, and dreams, every painting is nevertheless distinct from the psyche of the artist. The creative process will not tolerate the making of facsimiles. It transforms whatever it touches.

If the idea of paintings emanating from the artist is excessively person-centered for some, then we can look at the reverse possibility and imagine artists as agencies of preexisting images. It is the process of intimate collaboration that forms the basis of our method and not a doctrine of origins.

Our sense of the creative process moves beyond the self-referential world of the person of the artist. We are interested in the things that come to us, move through us, and influence us. The making of a painting is an expression of that aspect of the psyche that changes, transforms, and constantly creates new life. The psyche is itself restructured in response to the influences of its own creations.

It is possible that the external forms of art do correspond with the inner environment of the artist's psyche. If we begin to think about the motivation of artists, it is natural to ask: Why do they paint? Where does this process come from? Do the forms say anything about the artist who made them?

I can say many things about why I make pictures and what I was feeling while painting an image. Whenever I look at one of my paintings I am able to describe something different, engaging whatever state my psyche is in at a particular moment. I can never make a final statement about an image since the two of us are constantly traveling in a context of change. All of the questions we ask, the stories we tell, and the feelings the pictures arouse enhance the psychological engagement of the image.

The paintings I make can change my life. Rather than revealing something about who I was when they were created, the images will sometimes make a statement influencing what I will become. As the images change, I change. I can never be sure which is having the primary influence on the other. Creation is a collaborative process and an intimate relationship between artists and their materials in which the participants continuously transform one another.

The skilled painter knows how to "feel into" the emerging image in order to help it *form itself* in ways that realize *its* potential. Even beginning painters are constantly involved in an effort to shape the picture as well as possible for its sake and not necessarily their own. The painting that comes into existence will affect the emotions of the painter, and sometimes this can be negative, producing frustration, dissatisfaction, or anger. These emotions influence the artist's next attempts at painting. The emotional history of the painter is one of many factors that contribute to the making of an image.

As a beginning art therapist I rejected Freudian analytic psychology and its diagnostic industry's assumption that the works of artists can be reduced to facts about a person's past. These judgments were based on a single, psychosexual theory of behavior. Years of studying the artistic motivations of children and adults have shown me that there are multiple motives for creative expression. In addition to observing artists' work, I have dialogued with them about their motives (McNiff, 1977, 1981). Attempts to unravel the labyrinthian dynamics of art's propulsion according to the categories of the reasoning mind— mine and those of the reductionists—will never replace the mystery with an explanation. If we achieved anything with our multiple motivation research, it was the correction of the tendency to assume that a complex and mysterious phenomenon can be explained by one theory. All of my reflections on the source of art confirm the inability of the mind to "explain" its origins. The phenomenon simply exists. Art cannot be isolated from its context and then used to support a foreign system of concepts. According to Jung, "the bird is flown" (1958, p. 199) when we attempt to explain the mystery.

Imaginal Realism

IN MY FIRST attempts to describe how the art therapy process works I used the traditional method of case study, and it took many years for me to see its limitations. The dissatisfaction started with the feeling that descriptions of what other people did would always be contrived. The case study is a construction, a secondary as opposed to a primary presentation of the artistic process. I began to feel that art therapy could not realize its potential as a depth psychology as long as it operated within case studies. It will stay "secondary" as long as it uses secondhand methods of presentation. Just as pioneering psychoanalysts worked with their own dreams, art therapists have to reflect upon the psychological aspects of their own expression. However, there are few precedents for direct interpretive engagements between artists and their images. The profession has largely followed the conventions of psychological case studies as contrasted to direct and personal artistic research.

Further, the explanations of artists can be dogged by the same secondary descriptiveness that we see in case studies. When we respond to art with art, however, we are given the opportunity to bypass perfunctory descriptions—those of the artist as well as of the secondary interpreter. When images interpret one another, every aspect of art therapy is engaged in an ongoing process of creation. Interpretation is revisioned as compassionate feeling, sensitive perception, and expression of emotions. John Keats felt that the "intelligence" of "the human heart" is the medium of soul-making. According to Keats, souls are not made until "sparks of the divinity . . . acquire identities, till each one is personally itself."

Research into art as depth psychology requires methods that enable artists to be psychological about their experience rather than depending exclusively upon others for the presentation of vicarious psychologies. Instead of staying in the role of making "unconscious" psychological expressions through their works, artists can begin to complete the psychological loop by reflecting upon the manifestations of psyche. Many artists have been reluctant to do this, fearing that once they know the nature of their conflicts, their muses will disappear. Feeling that "the image speaks for itself," they have also been reluctant to get involved with explanations and conceptual interpretations, which interfere with the viewer's imagination of the image. As Vincent Ferrini said to me, "I stoop to explain."

Artists instinctively avoid language that does not respond to the image and to the creator's personal relationship with the muse.

These problems are mitigated when we shift to a psychological perspective which insists that a picture can never be explained or labeled with absolute finality. Experience in art therapy has repeatedly shown that meditation on the significance of the image for its maker and/or interpreter furthers, rather than obstructs, the making of art. Meditations on images and talking about them amplify their expression and help us to see things that we did not see before.

Our belief that soul reveals itself through the reflections of the artist adds yet another genre of interpretation, close to autobiography yet beyond the scope of persons merely talking about themselves. It is the soul that tells its story through the artist. This idea of the soul expressing itself makes it necessary to reconsider the notion that everything an individual artist makes is a self-portrait.

I am asked, "Is the painting you draw of the animal a self-portrait?"
"Yes and no."

Yes, everything that I make has an autobiographical "aspect" to it. All figures appearing in my paintings are expressions of my imaginal experience and therefore offer a self-portrait of psychic life. But autobiography and self-portraiture themselves open us to the realization that something is acting through us and that "the soul's deepest will is to preserve its own integrity" (Lawrence, 1972). Primary and individualized methods of reflecting take us into ourselves and ultimately to the soul process that moves through us and tells the story of *its* life—fiction joins biography and autobiography as modes of interpretation. However, fiction is not an "unreality." It is a different reality, the movement of imagination—what we call *imaginal realism*, a direct presentation of the life of imagination by the person who is experiencing it. So self-portraiture is paired with the portraiture of imagination. The two are inseparable.

My students have been my teachers in the formulation of these principles. For over twenty years I have had the opportunity to watch art therapy graduate students psychologically engage their art. Although these students are keenly interested in the art made by the people with whom they work in clinics, hospitals, and schools, their deepest and most formative training in the therapeutic use of art has taken place when they involve themselves in the process and when they let the soul speak for itself. They learn how to navigate the terrain, and this prepares them to be helpful to others. The history of psychoanalytic training affirms the primary role of educational analysis. Jung said that a method or a psychological principle is not understood until it is experienced. He felt that we have to know situations "from inside."

The privacy of the work done by students did not lend itself to public presentation. I was also concerned about the sanctity of the relationships that people establish with their images and how this is desecrated when the experiences are "used" by others to fortify their point of view or theory. This was the beginning of my sense that we had to find alternative modes of presentation that are consistent with the experiences upon which we reflect. If I were to "describe" the things that were happening in my studios, I would be again speaking "secondhand," as in the case study. I concluded that the only way to present the primary work is to follow the example of my students and show my pictures rather than just describe those of others. By leaving the conventions of description in psychology and in art, I would venture into a mode of presentation that corresponded to the way in which the work was done.

If art therapy is to move toward primary interpretive interactions between artists and their pictures and away from the secondary and vicarious interpretations of other people, we have to establish models for this type of engagement and inspire others to participate. My graduate students and the participants in my studio retreats have led the way and they have stimulated me to become involved. I may have had some ideas that supported their expression, and I may have been involved with convening the events where the work is done, but ultimately soul emerges on its own and initiates new aspects of the artistic experience.

In *Depth Psychology of Art* (McNiff, 1989) I took a step toward demonstrating how artists can respond directly to their pictures. I presented my interpretive reflections on paintings that I made over the course of a year in different art therapy studios. I feared that readers would say, "Why is he showing his own art? In art therapy we work with other people and we present what they do." I see now that the process was a demonstration by an art therapist engaging expression's movements and images and not just himself. It is the archetype of art therapy that emanates through us when we live the discipline and establish a camaraderie with our patients and images.

During the writing of that book, methods of dialoguing with images were taking shape. In art therapy we were meditating on images and allowing them to speak to us. We trusted the images and followed their lead. They expressed the nature of the work.

Dialogue complements the narrating ego with its stories and descriptions. It is more direct, intimate, and to the point. Dialogue is alive, and I feel more alive when I shift to this way of talking. Others have told me that the same thing happens to them. Interaction and surprise characterize dialogue as contrasted to descriptive statements. Anything can happen. Images speak to us and through us. Expression is free to move as it pleases and is not constrained by the logical sequence and distance that a discursive statement demands. Image dialogue is a dramatic language that transforms the way we look at art.

As a college student reading Plato, I missed the message that lay in the process of presentation—that is, in *dialogue*—as well as in the ideas of his philosophy. Dialogue assumes interaction between differences. It permits contradictions, conflicts, sudden shifts, vital exchanges, and there is no need to follow a single thesis. As the basis of psychotherapy, dialogue becomes a spontaneous and lively drama corresponding to the movements of psyche.

In addition to working with my graduate students and art therapy colleagues, I have been able to work with James Hillman in furthering the process of dialoguing with images. He has been a constant guide in the process of distinguishing our artistic expressions from ourselves as artists and appreciating them in accordance with Keats's vision, as "sparks of the divinity," "each one . . . personally itself." In the presence of Hillman I repeatedly catch myself in self-referential habits of perception and gradually open to a polymorphic view of the inner world where the ego steps aside and watches the play.

In practicing self-inquiry through art, I realized that I was not revealing "myself" as much as I was enacting dramas of my inner life with its varied characters. The notion of an "inner self" turned out to be a fantasy, a concept attempting to consolidate the diversities into an illusion of unity. As I looked inside and created pictures, stories, and confessions, I experienced many things but I did not find a person hiding from the world. The process of making pictures without following a theory or plan circumvented the linear thinking of self-presentation and stimulated a daimonic theater where multiple characters and varied themes appeared. The inner search is closer to Dionysian dramaturgy than a hunt for missing persons or holy grails.

In his book *Healing Fiction* Hillman shows how we unconsciously operate within a particular literary genre when attempting to describe inner life. Using the "disguise" of empiricism and writing behind this "mask," Freud created "pure fictions" and adapted every life situation to the single Oedipal plot. Because of this inability to embrace diversity, his theory "fails poetically." Yet Freud's bold and sweeping inquiries have had an unparalleled influence on twentieth-century consciousness. In declaring that the stories need to be "doctored," Hillman offers a revolutionary basis for art therapy based on the subliminal artistic identity of Freud, the reality of imagination, and the fact that life does imitate art. "Successful therapy is thus a collaboration between fictions, a revisioning of the story into a more intelligent, more imaginative plot . . ." (1983, pp. 18–19). Hillman suggests consideration of the "picaresque mode" in which a "central figure does not develop (or deteriorate), but goes through episodic, discontinuous movements . . . success and failure is measured by the flavor of daily experiences" (ibid., p. 18). Therapy is reimagined as a crafting of realities within the disciplines of artistic media or the interactive art of psychotherapy.

The linear narrative that I tell about how I construct a picture, or remember a dream, is one perspective on the action. Exclusive reliance on narrative generates what Hillman calls "ego theory." He says that " 'history' must be yoked to chronicity, but psychic realities, as both Freud and Jung insisted, do not follow laws of time" (ibid., p. 12). Joyce's *Ulysses*, like Homer's prototype, demonstrates how art generates formal structures corresponding to the varied movements of imaginal reality, which shift between narrative, dreams, fantasy, myth, meditation, action, description, dialogue, and other poetic expressions. Hillman's revisioning is to psychology what Joyce's *Ulysses* was to literature. Art as medicine instinctively follows the *Ulysses* archetype of episodic action and diverse forms of expression, spanning years or a single day.

My early inclinations toward total artistic expression, *Gesamtkunst-werk*, were viewed by some colleagues as a provocative crossing of disciplines that challenged the ruling sovereignties. By contrast, Hillman's post-Jungian archetypal psychology pairs art and therapy and embraces the intricacies of each: "This diversity of answers betrays a premise of archetypal psychology, that is, there are a multiplicity of answers to all major, archetypal, sorts of questions" (ibid., p. 57). When I paint and interact with the images, the discourse involves an interplay among my spontaneous inclinations. I enter the imagination of the picture and the stories that emerge from them. As Hillman says, "they are not concerned with 'me' but with the world they inhabit and which refers to me, the introspector, only obliquely" (ibid., p. 58).

Art's medicine is an activation of the procreative and varied forces of archetypal imagination within our personal lives. Hillman describes how the scope of Socratic self-inquiry has been expanded. The injunction at Delphi, "Know Thyself," is extended to knowing the many figures within ourselves.

> Before Freud, knowing thyself in psychology meant to know one's ego-consciousness and its functions. Then with Freud, Know Thyself extended to mean knowing one's past personal life, a whole life recalled. But after Jung, Know Thyself means an archetypal knowing, a daimonic knowing. It means a familiarity with a host of psychic figures from the geographical, historical, and cultural context, a hundred channels beyond my personal identity. (Hillman, 1983, pp. 62–63)

When I speak about this notion, people often ask, "And how does this 'daimonic knowing' of myriad inner figures help the world? What is the relation of this introspective imagination to others?" Some find my reply—that this knowing leads to sympathy for others—to be soft, Romantic, and indecisive.

Vigorous, disciplined, and imaginative sympathy with the life situations of people, cultures, and inner characters outside my immediate frame of reference is a radical political perspective. It counters the often brutal ax-grinding that "well-intentioned" reformers inflict on others with their righteous ideology and singularity. Sympathy supports not vacillation but direct and imaginative action based on the specific nature of a situation. Art compassionately immerses itself in events while maintaining its flexibility of movement.

I understand the conservative, no-frills type who says that looking into himself is a waste of time. But he errs in thinking that the sole purpose of these inquiries is to benefit the people who do the looking. They look also for the sake of those with whom they interact. If I am aware of my feelings and the unconscious attitudes through which I view the world, I am more likely to be sensitive to others.

This approach is based on the morality of interplay, on a compassionate and disciplined study of other cultures and points of view. Reflection on the other will be experienced as condescending charity if it is not accompanied by sincere personal expression. The other says to me, "Tell me what you are going through, and that will be more helpful than telling me what to do. Give me an account of the conditions of your life, your wounds, the things with which you struggle and those that bring delight. I want to hear the longings of your soul, honest emotions, and not advice."

These are the politics of confession rather than concealment, overt expression rather than covert operations, sympathy rather than opposition.

Muriel Rukeyser called for the poetics of "total response" involving "confession to oneself made available to all. This is confession as a means to understanding, as testimony to the truths of experience as they become form and ourselves. . . . And the witness receives the work, and offers a total response, in a most human communication" (quoted in Jones, 1985, pp. 33–34).

People who fear going mad keep their distance from imagination. They say, "This commitment to imagination promotes craziness and a quagmire of feelings."

I reply, "The feelings and imaginal realities are here, whether or not we are aware of them."

A gifted painter in one of my studios was reluctant to go further into the painting process. She said, "I am afraid of being overwhelmed. I will lose my balance."

I spoke about how the natural course of the theme she was living might be a process of destruction. By letting the process run its course she would feel more intact than if she continued to oppose it. She was making a series of pictures of cabinets and said, "I am afraid of being lost in the chaos of cabinets inside cabinets."

"Go to the next cabinet," I said, "and be with it. The feeling is telling you in its emotional way to move on to the next picture and stay with the particular thing that you are doing. As long as you are in contact with the immediate environment, imaginal and physical, there will be no chaos. Craziness comes when you try to be somewhere other than where you are, where you turn against the soul's intentions."

Another person in our studio said, "What do I do with the patient who is afraid that the pictures will come through him and he will have no control, no power, and be overwhelmed by them?"

"All we can do is stay with each one as it appears. The feeling of being overwhelmed is like hyperventilating and losing the rhythm of your breath, which gets ahead of you. The artist is the maker of the picture, and imagination needs the interaction with him in order to appear. If you can watch the interplay while it is happening, you will not be overwhelmed. Imaginal reality is always situated in an actual experience, a specific image, an immediate reality."

Artist and Angel

No one of them has any being just by itself . . . but that it is in
their intercourse with one another that all arise in all their variety
as a result of their motion. . . . For there is no such thing as an
agent until it meets with a patient, nor any patient until it meets
with its agent. Also what meets with something and behaves as
agent, if it encounters something different at another time, show
itself as patient.

The conclusion from all this is . . . that nothing *is* one thing just
by itself, but is always in process of becoming for someone.

. . . the pair of us—I who am acted upon and the thing that acts on
me.

—SOCRATES in Plato's *Theaetetus* (Hamilton and Cairns, 1961)

IF WE IMAGINE paintings as a host of guides, messengers, guardians, friends, helpers, protectors, familiars, shamans, intermediaries, visitors, agents, emanations, epiphanies, influences, and
other psychic functionaries, we have stepped outside the frame of
positive science and into the archetypal mainstream of poetic and
visionary contemplation. This list corresponds to functions performed
by figures we know as angels. My reflections on the angelic aspects of
art are informed by the writings of Henry Corbin, a scholar of Islamic
religion who has inspired post-Jungian archetypal psychology. Corbin
himself has come as an angel to guide and support this leap into
imagination.

The idea of approaching artistic images as angels is a natural extension of the practice of dialoguing with paintings. Talking with pictures
has emerged from the dramatic tradition of psychotherapy and from
our tendency to approach images within the more general context of

the literary imagination. Angels are compatible with our reluctance to perceive artistic images exclusively as expressions of the nature of the artist who made them. We see the artist as someone who helps the image express *its* nature, and this orientation corresponds to the traditions of angelology.

When I was discussing this principle with a graduate student from Norway, she told me about an actor friend who was playing Peer Gynt and who said to her before a show in Oslo, "I wonder how he will express himself tonight."

Through performance the idea, archetype, or angel of Peer Gynt appears in an ongoing process of emanations. Just as Peer Gynt needs the human being to become physically manifest, actors need angels desiring to come through them. The artist enters the imagination of the creation.

The inspiration need not be restricted to "large" cultural figures like Peer Gynt. The feeling that wants to come through may take a personal and idiosyncratic form. Even lines, gestures, colors, and shapes can have an angelic existence. Artists are thus instruments of these manifestations.

But do the musicians, poets, dancers, actors, and painters express traces of themselves during the interaction?

Yes, of course. Creation is an interplay among the artist, the feeling, and the material. The resulting expression embodies their collaboration. This "group" interaction cannot be reduced to speculations about one participant. The interpretive reductionism of our twentieth-century psychologies, in which pictures are viewed as EKGs of the artist's emotions, signifies the loss of the angel. The psychic figures who accompany us in dreams and other imaginal expressions are perceived as parts of ourselves. We are left with the fantasy of living within ourselves rather than within imagination.

The person who has meditated on an artistic image and who has entered into a deep psychological dialogue with it has little difficulty looking at paintings as angels. The experience of dialogue affirms the painting's existence as a living, expressive phenomenon. We are touched and surprised by the things it spontaneously says to us. The angel is a living figure who exists as an intermediary between visible and invisible worlds and who brings attitudes of reverence, safety, and compassion to art therapy.

I am not speaking about the angel as an apparition that literally comes to people in the physical world. I am an artist reflecting on inner movements and do not wish to present myself or my colleagues as "psychics" who have special powers of communicating with spirits. Our sensibilities are nothing but the extraordinary resources of the ordinary imagination.

The artistic angel is not presented as psychic evidence of the spirit's existence. The imaginal realm is forever distinct from the explaining mind. Different worlds do interact: as Woody Allen says, "There is no question that there is an unseen world. The problem is, how far is it from midtown and how late is it open?" One world can never be contained within the context of the other.

Our sense of the angel in art therapy is poetic, personal, and practical. Even the most unmystical art therapist approaches paintings as messengers from the inner world. The person who is analyzing drawings of houses according to a diagnostic handbook may not be using the language of the angels, but the fundamental angelic function of the image is being maintained unconsciously. The picture is a spontaneous emergence from another realm, which carries messages for people operating in the sphere of human reason and psychological systems. Methods of interpretation focusing on what the artist "does *not* say" similarly affirm the presence of influences that live in an intermediate realm. Human theories might change, but archetypal functions continue.

The diagnostic approach is typical of clinical methods that do not look at themselves within the broader tradition of interpretation. There is an attachment to the idea of the picture acting as an intermediary delivering messages between worlds. Diagnostic interpreters are so concerned with attaching labels and reaching conclusions based upon the perspectives of their psychologies that they do not cultivate the relationship with the image and the internal drama that it invites. They take the message as though it were generated by a fax machine. Our free-spirited angels will never submit to labels that nail them down. It is their nature to awaken the soul and help it to contemplate itself through intermediaries— dreams, visions, feelings, paintings, music, poems, dance, objects, nature, animals, and even other people.

The angelic perspective approaches paintings as tangible and personal figures that influence the lives of people who meditate on them. Through contemplation I enter the world of the painting and its angels who arouse imagination, offer assistance, console, evoke feelings, or inspire me to paint again.

Henry Corbin described the relationship between the person and the image, or angel, as "an archetypal dimension because it grounds every being in another self which keeps eternally ahead of him" (1983, p. 118). The angels, like paintings, are themselves in a condition of ongoing multiplication, and far from being "fixed" forms, they are "always sending out another Angel ahead of themselves" (ibid., p. 133). We follow the lead of the image. Our methods in art therapy are *responsive* to the actuality of a painting that comes through our hands and thus precedes reflection. The process of making and responding to images is an ongoing metamorphosis.

Corbin felt that in "every reality it is possible to discern a person" (ibid., p. 137). This process of personifying locates us within a dramatic psychology where everything has the potential to speak through the agency of imagination. As art therapy becomes part of a dramaturgy, as contrasted to the conventional tendency to locate it within behavioral science, and as the pictures and aspects of pictures exercise their ability to speak, the process parallels the functioning of angels. In Western history the arts have cared for the angels and saved them from extinction. The angels, like the arts, live outside the rules of reason. These movements do not oppose or challenge reason. They express different needs of the soul.

Angels accompany imagination wherever it flourishes and wherever there is a responsiveness to its emanations. The process that we describe as art can be imagined as the survival, or contemporary emanation, of the angels who have migrated to the hospitable habitats of artists and poets. Corbin felt that the "influx" of imagination is equally available to all, although "whoever has in himself the aptitude to receive this influx receives it; he in whom this aptitude is absent does not receive it" (1988, p. 289).

The influx maintains its place unconsciously in the average person's life. Homes are unwittingly constructed as sanctuaries for familiar spirits. When we fill our houses with paintings, personal objects, family photographs, music, and other creative expressions, we are enveloping daily life in the plurality of angels.

Anyone who insists that imagining angels is a form of madness has not distinguished psychosis from healthy imaginal life. People suffering from psychosis are flooded with repressed figures and voices.

Confusion ensues because psychic figures are experienced as literal presences and cognition loses it ability to differentiate. We intensify the madness by denying the existence of these figures while simultaneously taking measures to eradicate them. Sick persons need guidance and support in making distinctions between imaginal figures and other forms of life. They need help in moving between inner and outer experience, private and public realms.

Fear of madness deters flights of imagination. We have lost the ability to distinguish varied states of being and reality, and tend to separate the real from unreal on the basis of positive sense perceptions. Poetic and imaginal reality is more varied. In the epilogue to his visionary *Recital of the Bird*, the medieval Islamic philosopher Avicenna writes about how people listening to his discourse will say: "I see that thou art somewhat out of thy wits, unless sheer madness hath fallen upon thee. Come now! It is not thou who didst take flight; it is thy reason that has taken flight. . . . How should a man fly? And how should a bird fall to speaking?" (quoted in Corbin, 1988, p. 192).

Our sense of the angel is not limited to images of supernatural beings, originating in the Judeo-Christian tradition, flourishing in Islam, and surfacing again in 1822, when the angel Moroni appeared to Joseph Smith in Palmyra, New York, and led him to write *The Book of Mormon*. Angels are agencies that continuously revive the religious imagination.

Cross-cultural manifestations of the figures we call angels and their shamanic forebears confirm the absence of consistent conceptions and categories. It is the nature of angels to avoid universal definition and to assume varied and radically individualized characteristics. They are specific and intimate figures of the imagination who manifest themselves in an eternal variety of forms or formless presences. They may be conceived as persons who emerge from the artist's imagination, as the force of creation that moves through the artist, as invisible objects of desire, and so on.

Mythic, religious, and artistic accounts of angels and related phenomena are as multiple as the figures themselves. Each representation is shaped by the image that the person or culture is living, in cooperation with the inherent natures of the angels. James Hillman says that while people want relationships with angels, it is animals that constantly appear in dreams and art. The animal images take on the angelic "functions" of guiding and restoring the soul's instinctual nature. Involvements with angels suggest an "attitude" toward psychic images that locates our individual expressions within the traditions of imagination.

We affirm the sacred revelations of the different religious perspectives on angels, and the suggestion that these personages are expressions of imagination is not intended as a dismissal of their reality. Imagination is a psychic reality. In the visionary tradition of Blake, Yeats, and others, imagination is viewed as a divine influx into history, a revolutionary and transformative force that regenerates vitality. Loss of soul is the fall from imagination in our individual and group lives. Once an individual vision is institutionalized and presented as fact, it has been appropriated by "regulators" and removed from the "divine" realm. We prefer to keep visions intact by contacting them through the meditations of imagination. Religions need not oppose the unpredictable multiplicities of the visionary imagination because the *mysterium* does not relinquish its essential and basic nature. It continues as the hypostasis of every manifestation. In our era when obedience to doctrine and control of the mind seem less significant than personal virtue, meditation, and the experience of creation, there is room once again for individual and independent angels who embody freedom of imagination and spiritual renewal.

I have described how the opportunity to practice art therapy came to me without planning. It presented itself, and I chose to respond and become involved with the shaping and practicing of the discipline. My soul is committed to experiencing a preexisting archetypal image and process in order to experience itself. Depth psychology has called this *a priori* image that we carry within our souls an *imago.*

I never felt that art therapy was an invention. It is part of an archetypal process that cannot be fully contained by our contemporary interpretations. Yet the depth of art therapy depends upon its precise individuation in the work of different people and upon the individual therapist's personal experience of the process. What we experience will determine what we give back to the work. The future of art therapy "depends upon how the soul understands *itself,* upon its refusal or acceptance of a new birth" (Corbin, 1988, p. 10).

Reviewing my history with art therapy, I can quickly identify a consistent force within me that encourages immersion in this discipline. In addition to offering enticements, the force creates irritation and unhappiness during periods when I have distanced myself from it.

For example, even when I leave the practice of art therapy to immerse myself in speculative philosophy or personal painting, there is always "something" that draws me back to engaging personal images within the drama of psychotherapy. Rather than think abstractly about "forces," "needs," and other concepts, I can imagine this attraction to art therapy as a guardian angel, a tutelary spirit, or daimon who guides my actions and helps me to stay in contact with the deepest images of my soul's desire. In my experience this guide is constantly changing its appearance and manifesting itself in the consecutive but related embodiments of artistic expression in painting, writing, drumming, and other forms. Individual art works are animated by the presence of the guiding image. Yet no single work can contain it completely because it is forever in motion and always going on to another manifestation, always completely present in its momentary manifestations but simultaneously ahead of me in its desire. There is no contradiction in this ability to be in more than one place at one time. The absence of unity and fixity reinforces the process of ongoing metamorphosis and creation.

The guardian angel is a survival of the Greek *daimon* and even Socrates, the avatar of rational discourse, imagined that he was guided through his life by a personal *daimonion*. The Socratic *daimonion*, an inner teacher or conscience, appears to be synonymous with *daimon*. My guardian angel, or daimon, is forever reinforcing my commitment to art therapy. The deep satisfaction I receive from sustained time spent in this work derives from the image that wants to be realized through me. Activities that do not contribute to its emanation are less satisfying, and practices of art therapy that attempt to "fix" the work in definitions offend the imago. When images in art are labeled, my reactions are emotional. There is a sense that something sacred has been violated. The initial reaction is instinctual, and it is followed by reasoned reflection as to why this is not valid. The angels of feeling are always leading the way. Instead of restricting angels to clouds and celestial domains, they can be imagined as emotions and reflections.

The Greek sense that the daimon is a person's individual destiny and character is affirmed by my experience. I have felt this figure as an abiding presence, even in childhood when it generated a sense of anticipation about the destiny of soul's actions. Every person has potentials that yearn to be released, and their realization depends upon how we respond.

The emergence of the archetypal image of art therapy requires my sustained commitment to its realization. The two of us form a partnership that is the basis of creation; artist and muse, shaman and power animals, Socrates and his *daimonion*, child and guardian angel, person in art therapy and pictures, and so on.

The presence of the angel is connected to the objects of our desire. I heard a song on the radio in which a man sings about how if there is a God in the heavens, He will be driving a silver Thunderbird. The animal spirits of the totem live on in the names of automobiles and in our longings for their powers and grace. The male deity of this singer's imagination is in an automobile rather than on a throne surrounded by winged attendants.

Corbin said that when the soul awakens to itself, it simultaneously visualizes its guide, its angelic *paredros* (partner) or *angelus interpres* (interpreting angel): "the soul that has awakened to its individuality can no longer be satisfied by common rules and collective precepts" (Corbin, 1988, p. 19). Through self-comprehension the soul "attains to the world of the Angel" (ibid., p. 86). It tells its own story and enacts a personal drama with the help of its guide, which accompanies the soul throughout its journey. This corresponds to the vision quests of the shaman, which universally involve the acquisition of personal methods and tutelary spirits.

In his treatise on Avicenna, Corbin articulates the essence of this archetypal process and soul's need for "an absolutely individual expression" of itself, its guides, and its symbols: "At the moment when the soul discovers itself to be a stranger and alone in a world formerly familiar, a *personal* figure appears on its horizon, a figure that announces itself to the soul *personally* because it symbolizes *with* the soul's most intimate depths" (ibid., p. 20).

Even Nietzsche, the champion of will and ego, demonstrates the presence of psychic helpers in *Thus Spake Zarathustra*. When Nietzsche leaves reason's discourse and speaks poetically, imaginal figures appear—the Persian sage as well as animal guides.

Zarathustra, or Zoroaster (sixth century B.C.), was Nietzsche's lifelong daimon of individuation. In her introduction to *Thus Spake Zarathustra*, Elizabeth Förster-Nietzsche described the book as "my brother's most personal work; it is the history of his most individual experiences. . . . My brother had the figure of Zarathustra in mind from his very earliest youth: he once told me that even as a child he had dreamt of him" (Nietzsche, 1917, p. 9).

In Zarathustra's prologue, he declares, "I need living companions, who will follow me because they want to follow themselves" (ibid., p. 37). Immediately after speaking "to his heart" about how he will sing his song "to the lone-dwellers," an eagle flew through the air with a friendly serpent coiled around its neck. An ecstatic Zarathustra saw them as *his* animals. He observes that it is more dangerous among men than animals, and as he sets out on his journey he says, "Let my animals lead me!" (ibid., pp. 38–39).

Since Nietzsche's Zarathustra is a figure without material belongings, the possessive reference to the animals suggests a relationship to them as psychic guides. As we have found in our work in art therapy, it is the actions of human beings rather than those of the psyche that are dangerous. Nietzsche confirms that when the soul declares itself alone and in difficulty, sympathetic and personal figures will appear. Once again the shamanic pattern presents itself.

Imaginal figures appear whenever we immerse ourselves in the speech of imagination and become a "stranger" to nonpoetic language. They are inseparable from the language itself. Creation can be perceived as shaping the potential images that live in the medium, in our individual imaginations, and in the space between the two. Harold Alderman maintains that Nietzsche "discovered his own voice, the necessary language which fit the nexus of his problems" (1977, p. 4) in *Thus Spake Zarathustra*. Theoretical arguments are transcended through this language and through Zarathustra's laughter and dance. Alderman supports his observation with a passage from Nietzsche's foreword to *The Birth of Tragedy*, written fourteen years after that book's initial publication: "How I regret now that in those days I still lacked the courage (or immodesty?) to permit myself in every way an individual language of my own for such individual views ..." (Nietzsche, 1967, p. 24). Expressive language appears as the angelic manifestation, and it experiences individuation together with the artist.

In *Zarathustra*, Nietzsche comes home to his soul and receives what Corbin calls the illumination of the angel who "announces a necessary individuation" (1988, p. 262). It is the person of Zarathustra who reveals and defines himself in Nietzsche's imagination. The author's daimon and lifelong companion, not the person of Nietzsche, becomes the object of a sustained meditation and embodiment that brings profound satisfaction. Even though Nietzsche's Zarathustra preaches self-actualization, the reality of the book involves the actualization of Nietzsche's angel. The angel "individuates himself" and spontaneously "announces the soul's attainment of its truly personal symbol, and the greatness of the Event resides there" (ibid., p. 259).

Nietzsche demonstrates how the arts concretize psychic images that reside in us *in potentia*, often outside consciousness. They give form to images of beauty and of dark realms that otherwise would not be assimilated by the artist.

The soul perceives itself in its meditations on images. By engaging the image of an emotion, we further the emotion. For example, the soul's concentration on the beauty of the beloved object "increases the ardor of its love" (Corbin, 1988, p. 74). Persons emulate the images of their desire and in this way bring about change. The image is a guide who goes ahead and initiates changes, which we internalize through reflection. By supporting the manifestation of *its* individual nature, we experience corresponding changes.

Citing Persian esoteric texts, Corbin says that "every thought *is* a person . . . every true thought *has* an Angel" (1983, p. 167). If we consider our pictures to be persons and angels, then we are contemplated by them. Everything is reciprocal. They adopt our characteristics as we take on theirs.

In our culture we perceive art as illustrations of feelings, representations of nature, and objects of meditation, as well as furniture, investments, signs of cultural status, and priceless treasures. So why not expand the spectrum by including angels?

That images are living things was brought home to me recently as I was installing a pole on our porch for an American flag that my wife gave me as a present. My interaction with the flag was full of childhood memories of my father folding an even larger flag that he flew on the Fourth of July. I recalled the series of rituals and taboos related to the care of the flag: display from sunrise to sunset; do not expose to inclement weather; never let it touch the ground; the honor of carrying the flag in a procession or ceremony; and so forth. Leafing through the brochure that came with my flag, I was stunned to read: "The flag represents a living country and is itself considered a living thing." This was not James Hillman writing about the animistic consciousness of the archetypal imagination. The living nature of images and symbols was being affirmed by nothing less than Public Law 94–344 of the 94th Congress dealing with "rules and customs" regarding our flag!

★ ★ ★

If we can imagine a painting imagining us, then we are in the visionary realm. What was once a gallery of paintings in which I sat alone becomes a place full of expressive "persons" who offer companionship through listening, watching, or imagination. Their medicines include intimacy, affection, and insight. Although they are physical objects that have a material existence in the room, they are also alive inside me, and they are participants in the soul's inner dialogues.

In my training workshops people frequently have difficulty "performing" image dialogues in front of other people. This is because the soul's dialogue is generally carried out in a visionary or meditative state. As we practice our discipline of image dialogues, the external environment is transformed into a place that welcomes and supports inner and personal speech. Poetic and private angels emerge through relaxed and spontaneous expression. Once we are relaxed, and if the soul is open, other people who have entered the imagination of the image further the dialogue with their questions and observations. The reluctance or difficulty that we feel getting started with image dialogues within groups is an indication that individuals, and perhaps the group as a whole, have not yet entered the imagination of the image. The persons and angels of a painting will not speak unless imagination is welcomed and nourished.

As we become comfortable with inner dialogue, the persons of our pictures may feel eager to speak. They will interrupt, cut us off, or perhaps they will be more polite and say, "Excuse me, but I am tired of your explanations. Why don't you let me speak for myself?"

A feeling or image arises and transforms the process through what *it* has to say. The desire to speak is itself a manifestation of the soul's vitality and its need to transcend explanation.

The reader might ask, "Who is doing the talking? The artist or the painting?"

Both. The painting expresses itself through the agency of the person talking. Dialogue furthers our sense of images as persons. In addition to personifying the picture as a whole, specific figures and the non-figurative qualities of a painting such as colors, shapes, and textures present themselves as persons who listen and express themselves. So each picture is potentially a community of persons.

Shamans tell us that the masks they wear are alive but do not speak by themselves. They require human speakers, and dancers if they are to move. Paintings utilize human speakers whose words emanate through the agency of imagination. But the pictures, masks, and dances also express themselves autonomously through their physical forms. The independent expression of the image is the basis of its being imagined as a person. Shamans who wear the skins of bears do not "become" bears. They use themselves as instruments through which the bear presents itself. Similarly, when I perform in response to an image in a painting, I do not become the image on the canvas. I use myself as an agency to present an image that lives through me, just as the figure on a canvas lives through the paint. The performance is inspired by the painting. The performance may be related to the picture or even imitative but they are distinctly different realities.

Many will ask, "Why bother talking with pictures? Isn't it obvious that visual images communicate without words?"

It is the nature of a picture to engage us through the senses rather than through words, but as we have discovered from the dramaturgic aspects of psychotherapy, there are many voices within that are unknown, repressed, afraid to speak, or unaccustomed to spontaneous and direct expression. Our perception of paintings is similarly limited. The pictures are typically far ahead of us in their expression, and our reflective faculties may not engage or even glimpse what emanates spontaneously, and often unconsciously, through the medium. When we paint automatically and with abandon, the painting and the materials we use are literally "mediums" between consciousness and psyche. Meditation on pictures and dialogue with them help us to see the image and enter its world. Art students know how the comparable process of the critique reveals the individual nature of the image. Discussion can further awareness, although it can never replace silent reflection.

There is always more than one way to look both at paintings and at emotional conflicts. The psychotherapeutic drama and the artist's critique each offer challenging alternatives to what we think exists in a picture or situation. We tend to become defined by our habitual life. As "the Wiz" in the movie *Taxi Driver* says, "You do a thing and that's what you are. You are the job."

Imagination can easily increase the scope of who "you are," but the expansion involves the ability to contemplate oneself as a plural being. This imaginal fluidity is not the clinical condition that we call multiple personality disorder. As I stated earlier, psychosis takes the imaginal condition literally and loses the ability to distinguish between psychological states and move freely between them.

   While the behavioral sciences have difficulties with taking angels and psychic pluralism into account, these elements are fundamental to the arts, and especially to poetry. In "Starting from Paumanok" Walt Whitman acknowledges "Living beings, identities now doubtless near us in the air that we know not of." His poem "There Was a Child Went Forth" suggests how experiences form a person.

There was a child went forth every day,
And the first object he look'd upon, that object he became,
And that object became part of him for the day or a certain part of the day,
Or for many years or stretching cycles of years.

   Whitman also intuitively grasped the archetypal couple within his psyche, what Socrates described as "the pair of us." In an 1848 notebook the poet writes: "I am always conscious of myself as two—as my soul and I: and I reckon it is the same with all men and women."

   The emphasis on interactive pairs in archetypal psychology parallels Whitman's intuition. Rather than striving therapeutically to unify the different aspects into "one," we encourage them to interact, or simply let them be and care for themselves.

   Even literary scholarship tends to interpret multiplicity as a "divided self" and an inability to achieve "integration." A recent biography of Whitman's "inner life" suggests that the poet's affections for his soul expresses love of self, which is an expression of "sexual defeat" (Cavitch, 1985, pp. 59–60). Poor Whitman, the person whom D. H. Lawrence extolled as "the first white aboriginal," the poet who sings his love for all the world, is interpreted as merging everything into himself and his sexual inadequacies. Whitman's imagination may have immersed itself in everything and everything in itself, but every word of his poetry celebrates the other that he is not.

   Whitman's poetry is more at home with Jung's psychology of "divine pairs" in which "the One is never separated from the Other." In "One's-Self I Sing" the poet declares, "The Female equally with the Male I sing / Of Life immense in passion, pulse, and power. . . ."

   William Blake similarly affirmed the necessity of "contraries." Hillman describes how mythological thought imagines through pairs rather than through opposition. He feels that gender is essential to thinking in pairs and that the masculine and feminine are not opposed. Hillman prefers "a 'hermaphroditic' consciousness in which differences are co-present, a priori, at all times" (1985, p. 177). He writes, "There is no *other* vantage point toward either than the other" (p. 171).

Thinking in pairs evokes the angel and its human partner, visibles and invisibles, spirit and matter. Our psychologies erroneously reduce these partnerships to oppositions.

Whitman pledges commitment to his angelic companion in "Song of the Open Road."

> Camerado, I give you my hand!
> I give you my love more precious than money,
> I give you myself before preaching or law;
> Will you give me yourself? will you come travel with me?
> Shall we stick by each other as long as we live?

And in "Song of Myself" the contradistinction of the soul from the reflective consciousness is clearly articulated: "I and this mystery here we stand."

The poet further proposes an equitable interaction rather than one based on dominance.

> I believe in you my soul, the other I am must not abase itself to you,
> And you must not be abased to the other.

> Loafe with me on the grass, loose the stop from your throat,
> Not words, not music or rhyme I want, not custom or lecture,
>   not even the best,
> Only the lull I like, the hum of your valvèd voice.

Whitman's poetry confirms the engagement of the imaginal other as a fundamental aspect of art's medicine and procreative satisfaction. In addition to the collaboration between "my soul and I," the interaction between masculine and feminine sensibilities has been one of the deepest and most productive forces in the history of art.

Vincent Ferrini said to me, "Walt Whitman and Emily Dickinson are the exemplification of art as medicine. Walt W. is the best female poet of these United States, and Emily D. is the greatest male poet. Whitman wrote long, flowing, laid-back lines, and Dickinson wrote solid, erect poems, loaded with seeds. Their poetry shows that they were healed persons through their art. If they did not engage the other in the flesh, it comes in art."

In her poem "Indian Summer" Emily Dickinson demonstrates the terse precision of imagery that Ferrini describes. Eros appears, veiled in metaphor and what the poet called "bolts of melody."

> Till ranks of seeds their witness bear,
> And softly through the altered air
> Hurries a timid leaf!
>
> Oh, sacrament of summer days,
> Oh, last communion in the haze,
> permit a child to join,
>
> Thy sacred emblems to partake,
> Thy consecrated bread to break,
> Taste thine immortal wine!

Through these compact and simply stated lines, the air is resplendent with ranks of spirits, a profusion of daimones.

The Daimonic Tradition

THE HISTORY OF the daimones within Western culture illustrates how our psychic functions and their "natural law" of expression have been polarized and suppressed. We have inherited a moral dichotomy between angels of light and darkness, the former identified with the good and complacent spirit and the latter with demons, passionate desire, and animal instincts. One form of psychic emanation is celebrated while the other becomes the suppressed shadow.

In the creative process, all of psyche's manifestations freely interact without *a priori* judgments. If we step out of the oppositional perspective, the angel and the demon are necessary partners in creation. Indeed, artists often fear that if their demons leave, the angels will go with them. Zarathustra, who proclaimed that there is no devil, embraced the demonized instincts: "I tell you: one must still have chaos in one, to give birth to a dancing star" (Nietzsche, 1917, p. 32).

"Demons" can be liberated from association with the dichotomy of good and evil if we reflect upon their ancestors, the Greek daimones, autonomous yet familiar figures who inhabit and guide human actions.

For thousands of years the daimon, closely related to soul, has been known as the movement or force of creation. Experienced as a personalized and intimate agency from which both angels and demons are derived, the concept of daimon is based on an acceptance that inspiration arises spontaneously during the artistic process.

Within the imagination of classical Greece, the daimon is the source of creative expression as well as individual destiny. It is useful to revive the word because, first, it does not have psychological or artistic stereotypes attached to it; second, it has a distinguished heritage within the poetic tradition; and third, it evokes many features of art that more familiar words do not.

Daimon is a divine power that reveals itself through action. Thus we see its relevance to our concept of creative process. "Daimon does not designate a specific class of divine beings, but a peculiar mode of activity" (Burkert, 1985, p. 180). Jung described how the daimon comes to us "from outside, like providence" and we are entrusted with "the ethical decision" (1958, p. 27). We choose whether or not we will cultivate the gift and enhance its flow.

The daimon is related to the Roman concept of genius and similarly serves as a guiding spirit. In our culture *genius* has lost its original meaning. To renew the notion of genius in art therapy, I have described it as the expressive style that is "native" to a person. Our objective is to support the emanation of the soul's individual nature, the genius of every person and thing.

The daimones of antiquity were connected to a particular person or environment. Like Celtic fairies, they lived in the trees, rocks, and waters, and the different arts or expressions had different guiding spirits. Because of these ties, everything in the world was seen as an ensouled entity. Jung felt that caring for the spirit required "nothing less than its daemonization" (1958, p. 111).

Although the daimones have been transformed into angels, guardians, and other heavenly hosts, their most vital manifestations in our positivist era have been as "demons." While the benevolent aspects of the daimon are viewed as chimera in our culture, the negative world of demons flourishes. Devils are commonly presented as animalistic and quasi-sexual figures. Whenever we are oriented exclusively to transcendence, the abandoned chthonic and sensual world becomes demonized. The earthly and imaginal instincts threaten the spiritual order which has not incorporated them as active collaborators, and the repressed aspect becomes a threatening shadow figure. Reason has made demons of essential aspects of soul because they do not fit into its moral schema, but the cultivation of soul involves an interaction with all of its qualities.

The daimonic view accepts the "I" and its moral obligations to society. However, it also accepts the autonomy of figures in dreams, paintings, stories, and performances, and it does not always share the ego's perspective on these multifarious and free-wheeling characters. All of our imaginal persons, including the pathological and unattractive ones, guide our actions. Artists need gnawing and goading demons to stir emotions and provoke primal expression. Their perversity is apt to stay around until we get it right.

In classical Greek literature the daimon has all of the qualities attributed to angels, spirits, muses, guardians, guides, companions, and familiars. John Rexine (1985) points out that the use of the word in Homer, Hesiod, and the pre–Socratics has no single English equivalent and cannot be reduced to one meaning. This actually contributes to its vitality because we must continuously reimagine its nature and its varied functions. I am attracted to the word's versatility and long history, which stirs the depths of memory and puts us in touch with the contributions of others who have meditated on the mysteries of creation. Hesiod identified daimones with the souls of ancestors from the Golden Age who were transformed by Zeus after their deaths into invisible guardians of mortals. When artists speak of the spirits of inspirational figures in art who move through them as they create, they may be echoing something close to Hesiod's ancestral daimones. The great artists of history certainly live on as guides and daimonic functionaries, taking up residence in the souls of later generations who have corresponding sensibilities.

Rexine says that the most frequent use of the word suggests that "*daimon* brings or is the *cause* of bringing upon man something that is contrary to his will, purpose, or expectations" (1985, p. 337). This aspect of the word reminds us of art therapy's ability to present us with surprising images. "*Daimon* expresses a wide range of meanings, from a specified god clearly known and described to an unknown, unspecified, depersonalized, divine power of great potency" (ibid., p. 348).

Walter Burkert also feels that it is not possible to give a clear definition to the Greek word *daimon*.

> *Daimon* is occult power, a force that drives man forward where no agent can be named. The individual feels as it were that the tide is with him, he acts with the daimon, *syn daimoni*, or else when everything turns against him, he stands against the daimon, *pros daimona*. . . . *Daimon* is the veiled countenance of divine activity. There is no image of a daimon, and there is no cult. *Daimon* is thus the necessary complement to the Homeric view of the gods as individuals with personal characteristics; it covers that embarrassing remainder which eludes characterization and naming. (1985, p. 180)

The daimon never takes on fixed meanings, because it is always moving. It is a formative power, creation itself.

The personal daimon is associated with the psyche of the individual artist, a familiar, in contrast to the agencies of nature and the influences of other people. Pythagoras considered daimones to be the same as the psyches of men (Ferm, 1945, p. 215), and for Heraclitus the daimon was a person's essential nature: "character is for man his daimon" (quoted in Hastings, 1928, p. 593).

Plato presents them as intermediaries between gods and humans, tutelary spirits. He considered the guiding daimon to be the most significant of soul's attributes, and at times *soul* seems to be interchangeable with *daimon*. Menander in the fourth century B.C. said: "By every man at birth a good daimon takes his stand, to initiate him in the mysteries of life" (ibid., p. 591).

To state that belief in autonomous psychic figures is a revival of "demonology" is to take these agencies literally instead of imaginally and artistically. That the existence of the daimon is connected to the imagination of the person experiencing it is beyond question. The process is real *within the context of imagination*. The sustained appeal of psychic figures affirms our need for their company.

To me, daimones are actual images, pragmatic actions, and inner experiences, a name for the inner sensibility or conscience that directs a person's life. Burkert describes how Socrates attempted to distinguish these real, psychological experiences from spiritism:

> When Socrates sought to find a word for that unique experience which would compel him in all kinds of situations to stop, say no, and turn about, rather than speak of something divine, he preferred to speak of something daimonly, the *daimonion* that encountered him. This was open to misinterpretation as dealings with spirits, as a secret cult. It cost Socrates his life. (1985, p. 181)

To me, "spiritism" is the belief that spirits are literally, as contrasted to imaginally, present—the literalization of poetic experience.

At the beginning of this century Jane Harrison (1850–1928) wrote about the mysterious and shadowy vitalism that infuses the *instinctus divinus*. Harrison believed that "the daimon is born of the rite and with the rite which begat him he is doomed" (1962, p. xlvi). She reconnected the image to the imagination from which it emerged, the mysterious and "dehumanized daimon." But as in the mystery cult of Dionysos, incarnated images pass on in order to make room for their successors. Harrison preferred the daimon to "fixed," immobile, and abstract deities that have grown away from the processes of death, resurrection, and new creation.

Group energy and support are essential to a daimonic environment, and most of my art therapy work is done in groups. Dionysian religion and shamanism both are based upon the group. According to Harrison the daimonic aspect appears when the participant within a group "is conscious of something in his emotion not himself, stronger than himself" (ibid., p. 46). The community of cooperative actors is an example of a group whose primary focus is the rite, the act, rather than the doctrine. As long as the rites are performed spontaneously in groups, calcification is impossible. The daimon of art therapy is not only a contributor to creation, but the guardian of the images' mystery and individuality, the one who deflects labels. We support emergent expression whose destiny is to appear, and die, and forever repeat this cycle. Daimonic psychology is always in transition and never consolidated around the life of a single personality.

The daimonic consciousness does not "develop." It is an innate sensitivity that we can exercise and condition like our bodies. It is something given to us at birth, our nature, the marrow of soul, and its absence is like a state of soul loss or a fall from grace. People are always mourning the loss of the daimon when they leave our studio retreats, which meet for consecutive days, but the experience of this loss, the lost soul, is an essential aspect of the process. It is one of many factors that help to regenerate the creation cycle. That is the point of it all—to do it again!

Before moving on to a free exchange with dreams and paintings I would like to review methods of interpretation that have been suggested in the previous sections of this book—meditation, storytelling, dialogue, performance, and dreaming. Although attempts at summary never encapsulate or define an artistic method, an overview will be useful for readers. It gives an opportunity to reflect on the comprehensive nature of the method as an abstraction, separated from its ongoing emanation in practice. The abstraction is a distillation from the experience of engaging images. It is an expression of the mind's inevitably incomplete and biased thinking about what has taken place. Our efforts to describe principles are based upon the realization that they will never replace the actual doing of the work which is always a step or two ahead of the reflecting mind. Experience also shows that methods are themselves in constant transformation.

Part Two

DIALOGUING
and
OTHER METHODS

Loquent Meditations

WITHIN THE ART therapy studio the interpretation of images is a group meditation during which we contemplate paintings by speaking with one another and with the paintings themselves. The deep affection that we have for the paintings corresponds to the devotional aspect of meditation. Interpretation is another phase of the creative process during which we respond to the art of picture-making through a creative discourse that has the freedom to follow diverse aesthetic, psychological, and spiritual possibilities. It is an art that we "practice" in order to become aware of the psychic aspects of image-making and of our reflections on the finished objects.

An advocate of classical spiritual discipline might say, "Speaking meditations? Isn't the purpose of meditation to move us away from the chattering mind? Meditation is wordless, silent."

Although compulsive talking and indiscriminate chattering are certainly obstacles to meditation, we do not have to dismiss verbal exchange. Speaking is part of our nature, and the nature of soul. Silent reflection is a natural way of responding to artistic images and has an important place in art therapy, but why exclude soul-to-soul dialogue? We can listen to the other and invite our different internal figures to express themselves. We can bring the reflective qualities of meditation to interpretation and combine looking with talking about what we see. Speech is part of the social dimension.

People are often unaccustomed to meditating on images and expressing to others what they experience. When they look at a painting, they assume that it has an established meaning, and either they try to explain it or they are baffled and unable to grasp its significance. We so often forget the ancient distinction between symbols and signs. Symbols and art works exist to express the unexplainable, and they continuously generate different responses within the same person.

Our method of dialoguing is based upon careful and sustained observation of the physical qualities of an image. What is it that we see? How do our perceptions differ and agree? What attracts the eye first? Where does it go from there? What do we overlook? We might begin by thinking only of physical qualities—texture, forms, lines, colors, contrasts, light, dark, edges, figures, backgrounds, placements, spatial relationships, verticals, horizontals, and so on.

This way of looking becomes a meditation on "the other." It prevents us from quickly labeling an image according to our frame of reference. We affirm the particular qualities that comprise its identity, the idiosyncratic traits that define the soul of a person *or* an object. The experience of soul is connected to the observation of specifics. It has nothing to do with generalizations, standard types, intellectual classifications, and habitual judgments. The person who looks into the soul of another contemplates facets of that person's being without judgment.

Dialogues with images are always based on visual inquiry. Having acknowledged the integrity of the other and its unique physical nature, we can become involved in more imaginative and psychological reflections with the understanding that it is the image that is expressing itself and stimulating our responses. In this way, the painting of the picture is a mode of artistic reflection that is followed by other phases of creation, and the context of each is clearly defined and its distinct character protected.

Creation Stories

THE METHODS DESCRIBED in this part of the book emerged from studios that I run for groups of art therapists. Although my early work as an art therapist was focused on severely handicapped people, my practice has expanded to the application of art therapy to all aspects of life. I encourage readers to adapt methods to the needs of their environments.

In my studios people instinctively tell stories about the images they make—the obstacles they faced, problems they solved or did not solve, unexpected happenings. I prefer to call these descriptions "stories" rather than "explanations" because the former suggests elements of poetry and emotion. The story is not necessarily a fiction, although invented and imaginary aspects can certainly further its dramatic and psychological impact. Storytelling is the soul's speech, and it is free to move between the realities of imagination and literal events.

The guiding attitude of this method is the treatment of images as ensouled. We approach them as we would a person, who similarly cannot be explained. A person cannot be labeled "dependency," "depression," or some other abstract notion. The same applies to animals and other creatures. Neither the lion who lives in the wild nor the lion in a person's painting can be reduced to "aggression." The more we know about lions, the more we see the unique and specific qualities of each animal. Labeling images betrays the absence of a deeper knowledge of the phenomena. They are unique configurations that exist outside the context of descriptive categories. As Hillman likes to say, "You would not say to the person in front of you, 'What do *you* mean?' " The label can never contain the image.

Telling stories about images maintains the phenomenological clarity of the different elements. Paintings, painters, viewers, and the words expressed in response to the picture are distinguished from one another, and the complexities of each are left intact. Labels and explanations assume that a painting contains the distilled nature of the painter which can be defined by a concept. All of the organic particulars are lost, and we are left with empty concepts lacking substance or body.

Our respect for mystery does not mean that we encourage obscurity. The stories we tell about images help us to see them with more emotional insight and visual precision. Stories elucidate the images and their psychological evocations while sustaining mystery. We affirm those aspects of the creative process which will never be grasped by the reasoning mind, but which nevertheless fuel the intellect and introduce drama to the interpretive process. Although it can be fascinating to continuously meditate on the physical qualities of paintings, the soul delights in the enactment of feelings and psychological tensions.

Stories are generally motivated by a desire to share the process of making the image. Although these narratives are another phase of art's emanation, they are reflective and historic, giving accounts of things that have already happened. They generally talk *about* the images and their emergence, as distinguished from the way we talk *with* them in dialogue dramatizing the living presence of a picture. During the storytelling phase of our work, people talk with one another, and the painting serves as a bridge between them. It is a silent third person whose presence stimulates people to engage one another. Stories stimulate reflection as they tap into the psychological dimensions of the image and the painting process. They involve the group in the discipline of meditating on the relationship of an image to the psyche of its maker. The story helps everyone in the group, including the painter, to become aware of the context in which a painting is created. It informs, inspires, and initiates us into the mysteries of the image.

As people take turns in telling stories about their process, the ritual aspects of the procedure are enhanced. Since we typically give all of the people in the studio the opportunity to describe their work, the group practices the art of silent response and affirmation. In our studios we have found that it is natural and important to acknowledge all of the pictures that have been created, so methods tend to be focused on the need to engage the image as well as the person. Telling creation stories is a *rite de passage* that initiates outsiders into the inner context of the image.

The leader acts as a guide to the process as well as its guardian. Conflict and difficulties do not have to be prompted by leaders. If the person feels safe and if the purpose of the work is clearly psychological, then significant themes and concerns will emerge naturally in their own time. People come to realize that the studio environment gives them the freedom to open at their own pace and without contrivance.

When we sit down to talk about paintings, groups need help in establishing clear, consistent, and safe rituals of interaction. Although our methods are always based on looking at the physical qualities of an image, we do not necessarily begin by viewing everyone's picture in terms of structure, color, and other perceptual qualities. Exercises of this kind take away the natural and spontaneous movement of a group.

People talking about their work need time and attention in order to establish the flow and psychological pace of their experience. I often encourage participants to take their time and give the story a chance to emerge; to feel what they are doing, and articulate what they are feeling; to let the listeners sit with the experience. Without this relaxed and sincere description of emotions, the experience stays on a superficial level.

Responding

MY ART THERAPY work is generally done in group studios where we continuously practice responding to artistic expressions and to each other. If I ask people who are telling stories to relax, then I want to protect them from elements of group process that threaten the sanctity of the work. The harsh self-critic is as disruptive to the process as the eager interpreter who jumps in with explanations or advice. Sometimes well-meaning people believe that the only way to support another person is through helpful comments, suggestions, or questions. In the beginning of our storytelling work I ask groups to withhold their responses at first in order to allow me to feel out the situation with the artist and encourage a full telling of the story. As a listener I try to immerse myself in the tempo, mood, and context of the person's painting and the story.

Artists generally want to hear comments on their stories and their paintings. I try to focus my remarks on the specific features of their work and refrain from introducing extraneous information. I might call attention to aspects of the image that were not discussed or encourage the artist to try experiencing the picture from a different perspective. After establishing a style of careful and sensitive response to the image, other group members are drawn into the discussion. It seems necessary to give beginning groups an opportunity to watch the process of two people working with an image and feel the emotional pulse of the interaction before bringing them into the discourse. Once attitudes of respect for the artist and the image are established, people quickly adapt to the context. They realize that the artist, and perhaps the painting, want responses from other group members that resonate with the tone and depth of the original story.

If I paint a picture with emotion, and tell a stirring story about the experience, I want to hear the emotional responses of the other people in the group. There is an interruption if I am talking from the heart in a vulnerable and open way and someone responds with judgments, explanations, or questions that take me away from the image. Soul is lost when the intimate relationship to the image is cut off and there is a corresponding loss of emotional relationship with other people involved in the process.

I have found it helpful to establish specific time periods within our studios for free discussion and criticism. This assures a group that we recognize the importance of ideas and will attend to questions.

Destructive confusion emerges when there is a lack of clarity and consistency within the various phases of our studio. For example, if a person is showing a picture and telling stories about how it was created, other group members are encouraged to tell what they experience when looking at the picture and listening to the artist's story. However, this phase of the work does not begin until the person showing art has made a presentation and feels comfortable going on to the group response.

The giving of responses is always guided by the principle of staying with the image, and staying with the person who shows the paintings. If a person strays far afield from the image, the group feels the loss of engagement. Irritation brews if the discourse is not refocused on the image. If we stay with the image and the artist showing the work, we maintain a sensitivity for what is needed.

Timing, sensitivity, precision, and sincerity are traits that we work toward in responding to one another in our studios. Strong, negative, or provocative statements support the group if the purpose of the expression is clear and acceptable.

When someone is showing a work of art, one response is to express feelings that the pictures and the story arouse in me. If I want to say something to the artist about what I feel about him or her, then this is a distinctly different type of response. If I also want to say something about how the group is operating at the time, then this is yet another aspect of response. All of these expressions may stay with the image and the immediate context but they involve shifts in focus. As important as all of these concerns are, they can work against us if we are not aware of how we change from one mode of response to another. The introduction of even an essential aspect at an inappropriate time can further confusion and instability in a group.

Here is a list of things that we definitely do not do when people are showing their art and telling the story of their soul: we do not talk about our problems with the group, another person, or the leader; we do not bring up something that the artist said the day before that is still bothersome; we do not ask questions about how we can apply the technique within another context; we do not question the value of the method; we do not make suggestions about how the painter can improve the picture. Before or after the personal work with images is the time to deal with any of these issues that are of real concern to the group.

The leader watches over the group, the images, and the environment. The paintings are shown, the story is told, and the group responds with the understanding that everyone will have a turn. This simple principle of making sure that everyone will have the same opportunity cannot be underestimated. The knowledge that I will be able to tell my story helps me to be there for others when they present theirs. Providing time for the different and essential needs of a group avoids a destructive crisis resulting from too many things happening at once. Confusion in groups typically occurs when basic needs conflict with one another for time and consideration.

Attitudes toward time are surprisingly significant within the art therapy studio. Time can be viewed as a "personified notion" that contains emotional histories. Being on time, having enough time, letting go of the past, concerns for the future, engaging the present, flexible engagement of unscheduled arrivals, patient postponement— the clock is the ultimate image of social regulation and it evokes our shadows of compulsion and inattentiveness to others as well as signaling the depth of our caring.

Talking with Images

WITHIN THE ART therapy studio, talking *about* images has led to the more intimate and imaginative step of talking *with* them. Talk *about* pictures is from the perspective of ego, which controls the contents of the discussion. When talking *with* an image, I engage it as a new arrival in my life and I continuously acknowledge and discern *its* physical presence. As a participant in the dialogue, it is less likely to be reduced to abstract generalizations.

Image dialogue is based on acceptance of the autonomous life of pictures within a world of interactions and multiple perspectives. The artist realizes that the process of expression is never finished. It is unending dialogue. In *Moby Dick* Melville wrote: "God keep me from ever completing anything. This whole book is but a draught—nay, but the draught of a draught" (1961, p. 149).

Artistic images are never fixed and are incapable of being described absolutely. Hillman advocates a method that constantly responds to what presents itself: "One works with the images that arise, not special ones chosen by a master code. . . . We reach too far, missing the daimones that are present every day, and each night too. As Plotinus said: 'It is for them to come to me, not for me to go to them' " (1983, pp. 78–79).

Dialogue is the method par excellence in its flexibility and in its ability to promote interaction among different figures and points of view. In supporting dialogue, the content is inseparable from the way in which it is expressed. Depth of emotion, compassion, and other feelings are transmitted by the mode of presentation, and are as important as the contents of a dialogue.

When I perceive the painting that I make, or the dream that I have as other than myself, I set the stage for dialogue. The painting might have something to say to me, and so I take on the role of listener rather than explainer. A shift takes place in art therapy when people leave the ego position and let the figures in paintings speak through them. These interactions may include both conversation and poetic speech.

In their art work, adults return to the kinetic and free styles of painting that characterize the art of young children before imagination is displaced. The same thing happens when they begin to talk with paintings through the imaginative mind. Fresh and intriguing statements are made. The person speaking is taken by surprise. A sense of vitality emerges from these spontaneous expressions, unrestrained by habitual explanations. Getting out of the ego voice and experiencing other perspectives are fundamental to conflict resolution, innovation, and productivity.

The process of talking with images is close to the free-association techniques of early psychoanalysis, which enabled "unconscious" expressions to circumvent the "conscious" mind. Freud described the artist as "leaving" reality to become immersed in creative fantasy, whereas we see the artist as a person who moves among different realities and psychic states. Creative fantasy is simply another reality. Freud's follower Ernst Kris described the creative process as "regression in the service of the ego." This orientation assumes that the reasoning mind expresses a reality than is higher than imagination. Our aesthetic emphasizes interplay among varied states of consciousness and "relativizing the ego" without making hierarchical differentiations. We value the ability to move among situations and experiences.

Realities interact in the art therapy studio when talking is paired with painting. Dialogue helps artists to see what they have painted and, ultimately, to paint better. Talking supports the articulation of the image, and as the characters of both mediums are deepened, the speakers experience sympathetic changes. Soul experiences itself as the dialogue. Words function as angelic helpers and companions to pictures and vice versa. Dialogue is carried on not only between speakers and listeners, but also between words and pictures. The philosophy and methods of "endless tandems" (Hillman, 1985, p. 177) permeate everything we do with art as medicine.

Dialogue's ability to make sudden changes and effortlessly generate insights has a subliminal effect upon participants. The practice of adapting to unplanned situations and making imaginative shifts in consciousness is internalized by the person. During the Italian Renaissance, images were introduced to a patient's imagination to stimulate changes. There was an emphasis on changing the images that lived within the person's psyche rather than trying to alter the biological conditions of mind. The Renaissance therapies of imagination suggest that we might be better off changing images, stories, and conversations than attempting to "fix" the organism that houses them. This image-centered orientation has fallen like a golden egg into the lap of art therapy. Art can once again operate as a "primary" therapeutic method in which the creative process restructures the images and interactive processes that shape consciousness. Too much attention has gone into changing the intangible idea of the self, too much pressure. We do not realize that by shifting the discourse, we actually experience changes in our persons. We do not exist independently of the things that we experience. We are shaped by our dialogues. They are agencies, angels of transformation. Changes in what we do strike to the depths of identity.

People need coaching and support in dialoguing with images, because they typically think it unusual and "out of character" or "childish" to speak with imaginary figures. Children, by contrast, dialogue effortlessly when given the opportunity. The adult has fallen from imaginal grace. Image dialogues are threatening because they are not part of our habitual mode of conversation. We fear that we will not be able to do it, that we will make fools of ourselves, that we will not be creative enough, or we question the legitimacy of the procedure. The ideas in our minds block the expression of new images. We think too much about what we are doing, what we should be doing. We are overloaded with information and fear the loss of what we have.

In English grammar there are three "persons" in the use of pronouns: the speaker (first person), the individual addressed (second person), and the individual or thing of which the person speaks (third person). Each of us exists in these three persons. The "person" changes in relation to the context in which it is experienced. I express myself; I speak to others and am spoken to by them; and we speak about one another. In contrast to perfunctory language that does not support imaginative discourse, poetic expression transcends the egocentric bias of grammatical construction. Within imagination, "things" are not restricted to the third person. In addition to having people speak about them, things can speak to people and people can address them as persons.

By simply stepping outside conventional grammar, our methods of interacting with images are transformed. Dialoguing with images helps us get a better sense of who they are, how they were made, and how they can influence our lives. By letting the image describe its emergence, we enter into the perspectives of the medium and imagination. We can contribute to the dialogue by speaking to the image and asking it questions (second person). The images also speak directly to one another through the agency of human beings.

Participants in our studios describe how they "feel" the conversations as discourse shifts into dialogue. The pictures and the experience of dialogue begin to act on our emotions. Paintings have stories to tell, feelings to express, complaints to make, and endless communications which expand the scope of our studio. If we view paintings as personified images, we identify with them in new ways.

By engaging pictures, and their different aspects or parts, as "persons" with distinct physical and aesthetic attributes, we keep ourselves in the artistic process and we do not replace images with psychological concepts. When we talk about pictures rather than with them, we are in the genre of opinion, and description. Talking with a person replaces monologue with dialogue; we can find ourselves in group situations where we talk to ourselves, or simply talk in the company of others without interacting and listening. Artistic dialogue encourages each person's expression but shifts it to a context of active listening and responding, in which the quality of the interaction is more important than making your point. We have found that this other-centered orientation helps individuals express themselves, since people make more of an effort to listen and support one another. These communication values can be liberating to sensitive souls that feel inhibited by pressures to express themselves in ways that are contrary to their nature. The forum of dialogue is continuously moving and adjusting to the individual styles and needs of its participants.

The Value of Dialogue

I AM ASKED: "What do people get from this work?"

I cannot make a definitive statement about the value of image dialogues, which is determined largely by a person's desire for immersion in the creative process, change, and new insights. However, my experience does show that image dialogues always expand possibilities for being influenced therapeutically by paintings and dreams.

I have found that people suffering from psychosis are living in states of perceptual fragmentation, withdrawal, and extreme self-protection. They are typically involved in autistic fantasies. Through image dialogues they make perceptual contact with a particular image and respond to it within a conversational context. Image dialogues differentiate states of consciousness and connect inner experience to external objects.

Outside the realm of psychosis, image dialogues deepen the creative process.

The dialogues help us to see more in our paintings. If I make a series of pictures of cows, I do not leave the specific images and conceptualize them as expressions of *my* femininity, "anima," the repression of the feminine, my nurturing potential, needs for nurturance, fear of nurturance, longing for mother, and so forth. These conceptualizations abandon the cows to the voracious and all-enveloping ego, which sees itself in everything.

In our studios we try to stay with the cows, enter their world, and look carefully at their distinct qualities. How are they similar and different? How do I respond to the feelings *they* express through their colors, textures, bodies, faces, environment?

Through dialogue I become sensitive to my interaction *with* the cows. Rather than try to explain "why" I painted the cows, I encourage them to speak to me and to one another.

We recall Gertrude Stein saying: "Rose is a rose is a rose is a rose." The same applies to cows.

Dialoguing with images is not always necessary. Cows being cows, they may not want to speak to us. Majken Jacoby, an art therapist from Copenhagen, enacted this desire for silence in our art therapy studio. She showed how entrance into the world of cows might mean leaving behind the compulsion to talk. The psychic cows may be emissaries of pastoral existence, artistic daimones who show us the pleasures of sensing without chatter.

In dialoguing with images we also articulate thoughts that we have about a picture but would not typically express because they might be offensive or reveal too much. Such situations in which a person says one thing while thinking something quite different are what I call "Woody Allen dialogues" (after a scene in *Annie Hall* in which the characters' true thoughts are revealed in subtitles). We are encouraged to speak with different voices and to present private reflections in our dialogue.

The Jungian tradition has consistently affirmed the value of dialogue with psychic figures. Mary Watkins has studied how literature's spontaneous and natural personification of characters parallels Jung's belief that the autonomous figures of the psyche "preexist" and "have a personal nature" before they come into contact with us. Quoting the poet Wallace Stevens, Watkins says that "the characters speak because they want to speak."

The value of Jung's psychology has little to do with "proving" the existence or nonexistence of autonomous figures. Psychic pathologies, wounds, and helpers all exist within the imagination his therapy activates. Jung's practice of "active imagination" follows the artistic tradition of encouraging characters and images to reveal themselves, to speak for themselves, and influence the person who contemplates them. This way of working contrasts to the "depersonification," "depotentiation," "reclamation," and "assimilation" through which the ego brings its "projections" under its control (Watkins, 1983, p. 23). In keeping with my art therapy experience, Watkins has observed how psychosis is distinguished by its "shallowness in the characterization of the imaginal other and marked egocentricity" (ibid., p. 26). She observes that "when one does not allow characters their autonomy, one merely projects from oneself, lending them one's own face. When one allows characters to speak, to be known apart from the self, then a depth and specificity of characterization develop" (ibid., pp. 24–25).

The experience of Watkins corresponds to our observation that the ego's routine descriptions of experience are superficial. The same applies to a psychological theory that fits everything into its view of the world. Once a person knows the theory, there will be few surprises. Our work is guided by artistic method rather than theory, which quickly becomes a creed when it is taught and passed on to other people.

The discipline of formulating the specific qualities of an imaginal figure, as distinguished from the self, is a therapeutic and artistic objective. While articulating the characters of imaginal figures, we are sharpening our aesthetic and emotional sensibilities.

In *The House of Seven Gables*, Nathaniel Hawthorne "meditates" on the aesthetic qualities of the house and begins to see it as a "preexisting" psychic figure. Hawthorne does not view himself as the one who is responsible for personifying the house. Rather he is a person capable of seeing and experiencing its personified nature, and its emotional history: "The aspect of the venerable mansion has always affected me like a human countenance, bearing the traces not merely of outward storm and sunshine, but expressive, also, of the long lapse of mortal life, and accompanying vicissitudes that have passed within" (1904, p. 17). Hawthorne's musing on the "seven-gabled mansion" demonstrates the precision and depth of the artist's meditation on the "imaginal other." The house is experienced as something distinct from himself and its physical qualities incite his imagination. There is an interaction that informs Hawthorne's writing:

The street in which it upreared its venerable peaks has long ceased to be a fashionable quarter of the town; so that, though the old edifice was surrounded by habitations of modern date, they were mostly small, built entirely of wood, and typical of the most plodding uniformity of common life. Doubtless, however, the whole story of human existence may be latent in each of them, but with no picturesqueness, externally, that can attract the imagination or sympathy to seek it there. But as for the old structure of our story, its white-oak frame, and its boards, shingles, and crumbling plaster, and even the huge, clustered chimney in the midst, seemed to constitute only the least and meanest part of its reality. So much of mankind's varied experience had passed there,—so much had been suffered, and something, too, enjoyed,—that the very timbers were oozy, as with the moisture of a heart. It was itself like a great human heart, with a life of its own, and full of rich and sombre reminiscences.

The deep projection of the second story gave the house such a meditative look, that you could not pass it without the idea that it had secrets to keep, and an eventful history to moralize upon. (Ibid., pp. 42–43)

Note the way Hawthorne suggests that certain images will attract the imagination more than others, and "the whole story of human existence may be latent in each of them, but with no picturesqueness, externally, that can attract the imagination or sympathy to seek it there." Yet Hawthorne challenges us by saying that "the whole story of human existence may be latent" within the plain and nonpicturesque structures of our environments. We do not have to rely exclusively on grand and elevated images. The fertile imagination experiences significance in "the most plodding uniformity of common life."

Art as medicine strives to establish imaginal sympathies with simple things that are taken for granted each day. Actually, the things that we find most insignificant and even repulsive can be useful objects for dialogue. They contain our shadows, dislikes, biases, intolerances, inattentiveness, and sense of superiority. Commonplace objects—machines, trash, run-down houses, gawdy constructions, poorly painted pictures, "eyesores"—carry potential for imaginative dialogue about themes that we overlook.

In our art therapy studios, people who observe others easily dialoguing with dramatic paintings of emotional scenes will often say: "What happens if I don't have provocative figures, mysterious architecture, tender animals, mythic environments, and labyrinthian passages in my pictures? Can I talk seriously with a painting that looks like a first-grader's? What do I do if I just paint colors, forms, or lines?"

These situations enable us to show that simple pictures, which at first seem unimpressive, can serve as sources of stimulating dialogue. People who think their pictures look like children's work might consider listening to what the image has to say about that.

The picture feels insulted and asks, "What's wrong with a first-grade painting? And isn't the first grade the place where you stopped making pictures? Maybe you have to go back to the first grade of your imagination, back to the fundamentals, in order to begin to paint. First you praise the freedom and spontaneity of children's art and wish you could be that free, and then you begin to judge your work as 'childish' and reject it. You sound confused. Whom are you trying to please? Why can't you enjoy yourself? Why is everything so serious?"

And for those who doubt whether they can talk to a series of lines or composition of colors, I will often make a simple line on a piece of paper and demonstrate how it can become the most important thing in my life at that moment. If I can immerse myself in the nature of the line, it will reveal "wonders."

When it is labeled "meaningless," the line says, "I just am. Why do I have to have a meaning? Why can't you accept me for what I am? I am a simple and humble line, but I have feelings and I exist. I don't ask you what *you* mean."

I can take the lines and colors seriously and begin to talk to them about their textures, their subtle movements, the way they touch and do not touch, the energy that they generate through their patterns. They might be pleased with this more careful and aesthetic contemplation and tell me so.

"Now we feel like you are really looking at us and not using us to ask the same old questions about meanings. You are not judging us anymore. You are looking and getting to know us better. We have a lot to give you, but you have to relax and pay attention to what we are saying."

Painful and difficult experiences are typically the raw material of art therapy, which assuages the sufferer by transforming irritants, anxiety, and distress into life-affirming creations. But people in our studios also need support in staying with their ordinariness and their banal concerns. A man in a Sante Fe studio told me that an "addiction to breakthroughs" characterizes many therapy groups. Graduate students at Lesley College in Cambridge have facetiously described implicit demands for primal tears and confessions in therapeutic culture. Beginners need help in realizing that openness does not mean that they have to tell their darkest secrets. Opening may simply involve listening attentively and describing how you are feeling at the moment.

A dog in a painting might say to a man seated next to a door that opens to darkness, "You are so busy trying to engage romantic and tragic 'depths' and conflicts that you leave the 'basics' to other people. When was the last time you cooked a meal, went to the grocery store? Tell me about how you choose your socks in the morning, how you make your bed. Why don't you show that side of your life to people? I bet you are thinking of some heroic adventure that will take place if you walk through that door. That door will lead you to the dishwasher, the washing machine."

And as the artist I reply to the dog, "You are nothing but a moralizer."

"And you like to argue," the dog replies. "Don't take it all so seriously. Take me for a walk. Throw a stick for me and exercise your animal nature."

In his essays on images, Hillman (1977a, 1978, 1979) interacts with a figure he calls the "protestor," who defines issues and "moves" the dialogue through spontaneous confrontation. Hillman's direct and challenging speech has influenced our art therapy methods. The strong, active, and confrontive voice emerges when a person begins to belittle a picture—"nothing significant," "just colors and shapes."

This disparagement brings the picture to life: "How can you call me 'nothing significant'?"

Confrontation awakens the artist's empathy with the image and its existence. The image might also draw attention to our unconscious devaluing, depersonalizing, and disassociation by speaking tenderly: "Please look at me as separate from yourself. Let me go, and see me for what I am. If you can see me as myself, you won't be so concerned with my saying something about you. You see me through your feelings of insecurity and inadequacy. They come between us."

Hillman's personifying is most penetrating when our statements wound or slight the image. He describes how the snake in a dream who is called a penis is offended, insulted, and thus unlikely to return. The image is not uncomfortable with sexual talk, but it wants to be seen for what it is. Personifying becomes the basis for standards of therapeutic ethics regarding the treatment and "use" of images.

Dialoguing with images takes place in colloquial speech. Our aesthetic and therapeutic stance promotes spontaneous expression and the natural and individual styles of speakers. We discourage jargon and the impersonal speech patterns of psychological systems. As with painting, automatism is encouraged.

The process of dialoguing can be introduced by asking people to reflect upon their inner conversations. A period of quiet meditation during which the artist experiments with imaginal speech builds confidence. During these solitary reflections the images speak without interference from performance anxieties. Private meditations are excellent practice for interactions with other people because they help us to become comfortable with the process of inner speech that characterizes every phase of image dialogue.

Direct questions invite responses and eliminate the need to be clever, creative, or competent. The picture is asked, "What are you feeling?" This simple inquiry immediately personifies the image, encourages it to speak, and moves the artist into the role of the picture's "speaker." Every image has a feeling to express, so the question brings emotion and drama to the conversation.

The artist might also ask, "What do you need?"

These inquiries are concrete, direct, and personal. There is a sense that the person cares about the image and wants to listen to its intimate expression. In responding to questions, the picture may tell us something about itself that is outside our preconception of what it is.

We discourage people from asking, "Where did you come from?" or "Why are you here?" These questions take us away from the actual picture and into speculations about origins, what Hillman calls metaphysical discourse. We speak with pictures as persons and extend the same social grace bestowed on another human being, encouraging compassion rather than interrogation.

After silently communicating with pictures, I ask people to practice with a partner who acts as a witness and confidant. Working with another person enables us to externalize the inner dialogue in a private one-to-one relationship that supports taking risks and trying out unfamiliar and potentially awkward ways of expressing ourselves. The privacy of the interaction helps participants to involve themselves in dialogue. Partners alternate functioning as "speakers" (the persons dialoguing with an image) and "helpers" who function as listeners and questioners but who are also free to speak spontaneously in ways that support the dialogue. These roles are not meant to establish a strict protocol or fixed therapeutic jargon. Every situation is different, and we interact through sensitive improvisation.

Our two basic questions can be applied to work with a partner. The helper addresses the picture, not the artist, and says, "What are you feeling? What do you need?"

The artist responds as the picture's speaker, and the helper supports that expression, talking only when it seems necessary. Both sides of the therapeutic tandem are exercised. The artist experiences the imaginal medicine and becomes familiar with its inner movements, while the helper practices the role of companion and witness.

Speakers are encouraged to shift perspectives and engage different aspects of a picture. This helps to articulate the plural qualities of an image and discourages clinging to a single point of view. The helper selects a part of the picture, perhaps an obscure figure or a dominant color that has not been addressed, and asks it how it feels, or invites the parts to speak to one another. One part is asked what it thinks about what another part just said, or how it feels about what the speaker said about it.

In one of my studios an art therapist found it helpful to ask her picture whether she could move it in order to view it from another perspective. This simple ritual of courtesy helped her see the image as a personified being and instilled a sense of respect and tenderness into the drama of the dialogue.

Entering the world of the painting often involves viewers in a complete reframing of its contents. What was once perceived as a "depressed" figure lying on the ground can shift to a reclining person who rests and makes contact with the earth; a frightening animal shifts to a "frightened" creature. These changes in perspective demonstrate ego's unconscious judgments. At times we practice reframing a painting as an exercise to further the variability of interpretations.

Partners can also help us express concealed voices. The helper asks, "What are you thinking and not saying? Is there something you are afraid to say, something buried and held back because it is inconsistent with your usual way of speaking, something hurtful or embarrassing?"

As in social situations with unfamiliar people, we start with inquiries that generate information and move to more intimate conversation as we become better acquainted. Artists meditating on an image open their hearts and describe what it makes them feel. Many find it more natural to begin dialogue in this way. It enables them to speak first as themselves. Speaking as the image is more difficult for the average person. But after feelings are expressed or confessed to the image, dialogue tends to move freely and imaginatively. When first introducing people to dialogue, I encourage them to speak freely to their pictures. Although we stress staying in contact with the physical qualities of the image in our dialogues, artists are invited to express their feelings to the picture, confess, or try out new ways of conveying emotion.

When I am working with a person for the first time, I will often speak as his or her painting, or as a figure within the painting, and this immediately engages the artist in the dialogue. I might ask the artist questions from the perspective of the image, or express feelings and needs, all of which open the soul to conversation.

These are examples of how to initiate image dialogues. Like talking to another person, the dialogue is not preconceived and limited to an established set of questions. Persons experienced with image dialogue incorporate the helper and the questioner into themselves. They establish personal styles of dialoguing and continuously introduce new elements to the method.

The skilled speaker works spontaneously within the immediate context without pretense. In describing "beginner's mind," Zen master Shunryu Suzuki said, "If your mind is empty, it is always ready for anything; it is open to everything. In the beginner's mind there are many possibilities; in the expert's mind there are few" (1970, p. 21). Beginner's mind permeates every aspect of art as medicine. The discipline emerges from constant "doing" and practice with an equally constant awareness of the folly of one person prescribing his method for others. Methods are always changing and beginning anew. The Zen tradition conveys the ancient wisdom of finding out for yourself, realizing that there is no single or true way for all people. Yet there is the realization that a discipline, "some particular way" of practicing is necessary.

> If you understand the cause of conflict as some fixed or one-sided idea, you can find meaning in various practices without being caught by any of them. If you do not realize this point you will be easily caught by some particular way, and you will say, "This is enlightenment! This is the perfect practice. This is our way. The rest of the ways are not perfect. This is the best way." This is a big mistake. (Ibid., p. 74)

When people begin to dialogue with images, there is typically confusion about who is speaking. Am I projecting my feelings onto this image? Is the image speaking through me? Am I saying what I think the image is feeling based upon my observation of its visual characteristics?

This confusion is productive if engaged as an aspect of the therapeutic process, dismantling routine order and stimulating the person to become more aware of different qualities of expression. Image dialogues help us to discover new sources of expression outside our habitual frames of reference. The process may be disconcerting at first because we do not understand who is speaking. This discomfort is to be embraced as an opening to new understanding, rather than experienced as a deterrent or defense against discovery.

Jung described how imaginal dialogue "is based on a deliberate weakening of the conscious mind and its inhibiting effect, which either limits or suppresses the unconscious." He also discovered these dialogues to be "naturally therapeutic" and a source of "rich empirical material" (1969, p. 190). He advised caution in introducing these methods to people suffering from thought disorders. In my experience, imaginal dialogue can actually be more effective than direct person-to-person conversation in some situations where communication is impaired by psychosis. The patient may be less threatened by the prospect of talking to a figure in a painting than to another person. Ultimately, therapists must adjust their methods to the particulars of each situation and avoid generalization.

Performance

A S WE CONTINUED to experiment with image dialogues in art therapy studios we discovered that the process of speaking, whether about images or with them, could restrict interpretation to spoken language. In an effort to exercise the arts more completely in responding to paintings, we began to interpret images through performance art and body language. The use of movement, dramatic action, voice, sounds, and changes in personal appearance and the environment enabled us to become physically incorporated into the imagination of the painting. Our beginner's mind, in the sense of our lack of dramatic expertise, opened a wealth of possibilities, and performance became one of the richest veins within the art therapy studio.

The performance dimension was a natural extension of our attempts to find more spontaneous ways of interacting with paintings. With performance art we are able to give the artist the opportunity to move with the image, to enact the impact that it has on the psyche, and to explore how the image affects the body. Through performance we move from two to three dimensions and consciously introduce the ritual aspect of art therapy. Artists are given opportunities to physically experience themes presented in their work—to wear the mask of the wolf and act through it; to enact the dark colors, movements, and unfamiliar spaces of the pictures; to make a ceremony of the water and fire in the paintings; to move through the labyrinths. By incarnating these themes in their personal actions, artists establish another type of sympathy, another dimension of experiencing and knowing the pictures.

Our performances are closely related to the visual arts. The planning of the stage and the interaction among actors concentrates on the presentation of an image, a series of images, or a changing image. The images of paintings are interpreted or expanded through the images of performance. The emphasis on presenting oneself as an image likens the performance to sculpture and environmental construction. Although movement, sound, and voice are encouraged, they generally serve the visual images of our studio. Holding a body position, moving slowly, and economy of expression deepen our engagement with the body, its unconscious memories, and its existence as visual presentation. This bias toward the visual arts is simply the *persona* of my studio work, a personal style that may not be shared by others. Indeed, different applications and transformations will no doubt unfold through work by other people.

I do not wish to suggest that there is a developmental progression that begins with painting, moves on to responding with stories, then dialogue, and finally performance. The performance aspect of art therapy is not necessarily higher or more psychologically significant than the other ways of working with images. Each tool has its distinctive merits. It is misleading to think in terms of superlatives rather than of varieties, each of which makes contributions to the process.

Although performance is generally preceded by the other activities (painting, story, and dialogue), we have observed that every phase of the creative work can potentially contain the others. For example, the stories that I tell about my painting can include dialogue with the images and aspects of performance. Our performance art always follows the painting of pictures and the storytelling process because we find it helpful for both the performers and the audience to have a preliminary understanding of themes. The paintings, stories, and dialogues establish the context for the performance, which may stimulate yet another generation of paintings. The ritual emerges directly from group experience with the assistance of an informed audience. However, this is not a "rule" of operation. It is just the way the method has emerged within the context of my experience. People with a primary interest in another art form will probably find it following another sequence and taking a different shape.

This variety is essential to our method of practice. With art there must be room for spontaneous creations and continuous transformations. In contrast to ritual procedures that are handed down without the freedom to change them, the artistic method encourages constant alteration. No doubt, my use of the methods that I am describing will change as fresh and intriguing possibilities present themselves.

People who respond to their art through performance in our studios report that the dramatic context brings the most complete release from debilitating self-consciousness. Theater offers clearly defined structures—preparatory procedures, beginnings, endings. The audience has a contributing role in making the performance an "event" to be witnessed. Their concentration focuses the energy of the performance and strengthens its transformative powers.

Performance activates a condition of concentrated "being." It is a ritual of full presence. If I read a prepared lecture to an audience, there is a distinctly different sense than when I look directly at people and speak spontaneously to them. A passionate and committed tone of voice will convey a distinctly different feeling than a monotone. Silence can be far more engaging than chatter in our effort to connect with others.

We generally limit performances to ten minutes to enhance focus. The participant senses that "This is it. This is my time." And the audience reciprocates with a corresponding attitude. Concentration is heightened by time restraints, which, far from creating inhibiting "pressures," stimulate creativity.

The brevity of our first experiments with performance was due to the need to accommodate fifteen or more people over a two- or three-day period. We also sensed that untrained actors working without direction would have difficulty sustaining longer enactments. Time limits not only addressed these practical issues but also brought many unplanned advantages. Even highly trained performers found that the brevity of the format served to intensify the work, largely as a result of its ability to hold the attention of the audience at peak levels of concentration. The sequential process of three or four performances following one another also demands that we do not saturate the audience and drain their capacity to respond. I have discovered that brevity, as in the haiku poem, helps to articulate the essential statement with a minimum of distractions. Brevity is also considerate of the audience and does not "hold" them through long and drawn-out performances.

People who take the risk of making performances want to hear the responses of the audience. Although this practice is not always appropriate for other forms of theater, our context calls for communication that furthers the well-being of the group. It would be contrary to our values and group tempo to present the performances one after the other without time to reflect and comment. We take approximately twenty to thirty minutes after a performance to contemplate the work. The audience gives comments and support to the performers, who listen without responding and then speak to the audience. Comments are generally restricted to expressions of what performers and audience "experienced" during the performance. Because of the ritualized manner in which this takes place, the dialogue between actors and audience is like another phase of performance rather than an evaluation.

The practical need to efficiently manage time generated yet another unplanned innovation. At first our performances were individual enactments, like the painting process itself. We originally experimented with making performances in pairs and groups of three or four in order to have adequate time for reflection and comment after each enactment. We were surprised to find that the cooperation that emerged through the performances deepened the individual work of painting. The performances gave our group studios another avenue of cooperative creation. Participants had another person with whom to dialogue during the planning phase; they stimulated and influenced one another during the performance; and they were able to share the work afterward with a co-performer. Once again, method is both content and objective of the work. The same applies to the process of dialoguing with the group after the performance. Different aspects of creativity are exercised through work with individuals, pairs, and groups.

Working together with one or more persons in a performance immediately presents questions of subject matter. Two people may choose to work together because their paintings express similar themes that can be consolidated into a single performance. Others will collaborate because their themes are antithetical and can stimulate dramatic tension. A couple may simply be intrigued with each other, or they may be the last two unpaired participants. In any case, interaction inevitably emerges into a performance.

Performances do not have to be planned around common themes. Some of our most stimulating pieces involve separate but simultaneous action. Simultaneity offers contrast and freedom from the pressure to be in complete sync with a partner, a way of working that often generates tedious mirror movements or anxious efforts to connect.

Our performance art is always a sacred theater. For example, in a Swiss studio, a Lutheran minister worked with a woman from Finland who was involved with shamanism. The minister had been painting large pictures concerned with free experimentation with color, texture, movement, the interaction of forms, and variations of marks made by simple gestures. His physical experience of paint was not focused on making figures. In his stories about the pictures, he spoke of how his life as a minister made it difficult for him to express the full range of his emotions, especially his negative feelings and shadowy instincts. His role demanded him to embody light and goodness, and did not give him the opportunity to engage conflicting feelings within a sacred context. In his paintings he moved with childlike spontaneity, and he did not judge the work as "childish." He was proud of his playful forms, dynamic brushstrokes, and vibrant colors.

In his performance the minister did not explicitly enact elements of his pictures. Cooperation with the Finnish woman stimulated him to go further with themes of free expression. Her paintings presented shamanic figures and rituals, and this became the focus of their performance. Their collaboration enabled him to enter sacred realms that were inaccessible in his ministry.

Throughout the performance she beat a shaman's drum in a simple, steady, yet driving rhythm. Her paintings were hung behind them, bringing the spirit of art into the enactment. She was wearing one of the paintings that the minister made on rice paper. An opening was cut for the head to pass through so that it could be worn as a chasuble. He appeared also wearing one of his paintings, with his face painted and his hair gathered together and tied at the top of his head like a samurai. The way in which the paintings were worn gave the impression of vestments, and this reinforced the ritual aspects. It was midnight and the studio was illuminated only by candlelight. While she continued to drum, he knelt facing the group and did not move, allowing the force of the drum and the energy of the event to enter him. He lifted both of his arms, began to move, and sang a deep, primal chant that continued until the end of the performance. His vocal expression reinforced her drumming and moved the performance into another dimension. In addition to demonstrating how the soul appears through the voice, his expression was particularly strikingly because his normal speech was soft and almost timid. The audience was stunned by the deep resonance of his sounds.

Other enactments have supported the banal and ordinary aspects of life, which also can be strikingly dramatic. I recall a performance in which a woman who always wore her hair tied into a ball turned her back to the group, untied the hair, which fell to her waist, and then brushed the hair for the remainder of the piece.

As in much performance art, the body is often a focal point of the enactments in our studios. In another studio in the United States, a man who wore a hearing aid in each ear placed a full bowl of water on the floor. He knelt and turned his back to the audience, took off his shirt, removed both hearing aids, and placed them on the floor on either side of him. The audience was struck by the high-pitched sounds that the hearing aids made, and many people for the first time were aware of the degree of his hearing impairment. Because of the simple structure of the performance, every movement of his body became significant. The lateral movements of his arms in placing the hearing aids on the floor were particularly evocative. The sounds of the hearing aids added yet another dramatic element. After kneeling without movement for about a minute, he bent over and washed his face, the sounds of the water contributing yet another dimension to the enactment. After washing, he carefully dried his face with a towel, which he had placed next to the bowl. The performance was completed by refolding the towel and removing the bowl of water.

The man's partner during this piece was a woman who entered the room in her robe, paying no attention to him, nor did he acknowledge her presence. Throughout the performance she stroked her body, massaging herself in a comforting way, giving the impression that she was involved in private reflection. The two performances went on at the same time and complemented one another beautifully without direct engagement. The actions of the performers were related through simultaneity and proximity alone.

The performances that I have described affirm the dramatic principle that "less is more." I tell our studio participants as they prepare for their performances, "The simpler, the deeper. Depth is on the surface. Move slowly. Don't overact. Pause and hold your positions so that the body becomes sculptural. Give the audience an opportunity to meditate on your presence. Present yourself and your environment as an image."

I discourage drawing the audience into the piece. This takes away their ability to witness, and it can create role confusion, especially if the audience is asked to do things that are uncomfortable or offensive. The performance can easily turn into chaos. A chaotic art experience may have its place, but it can also be problematic. If I am drawn into a piece in this way, I lose my role as leader. It is not the loss of authority that concerns me but my inability to watch the process and protect people and the performance itself.

The discipline of performance art can include all aspects of life. At the Lesley College Graduate School, a woman whose art involved sewing delivered her paper for our course in a package covered with Belgian linen which she had sewn. It was an elegant object, with patterns of thread stitched onto the linen. She took me by surprise and made the routine process of leaving a term paper at a professor's office an art event. I enjoyed looking at her art work as it sat on my desk. It transformed the environment of the office and my conception of work. It was a charm that helped me become more aware of how art can apply to life. I was left with many decisions that drew me into the ritual of her art. "How will I open the package? When will I do it? Can I open it? Will I take away its mystery by opening it?"

Performance art aligns the art therapy studio with the efforts of avant-garde artists to remove boundaries between art, life, and the ongoing process of imagination—as do our image dialogues. Art as medicine returns the image to its archetypal role as a source of power within an interdependent environment. My student's presentation of her paper as an art work demonstrates how simply this can be achieved. The art object was functional, yet it was also a magical object that changed its surroundings.

Art therapy's conception of art historically has been closer to the conventional notion of the object as a record of an experience that has already taken place. The image has been seen as an extension of the artist's consciousness rather than as a living thing that influences its milieu, as an illustration rather than an agent of transformation. But as Allan Kaprow said in *Assemblage, Environments and Happenings* (1965, p. 156), painting then lost its archetypal function as a "power" and "*stood* for experience rather than *acting directly upon* it." Kaprow felt that "the line between art and life should be kept as fluid, and perhaps indistinct, as possible" (pp. 188–189).

The presentation of the body as an image helps eliminate the separation of the art work from its environment. Costumes, together with the archaic practice of painting and decorating the body, bring yet another trace of shamanic practices. Artists enter, move within, and leave the environment of the performance.

As temporal events, performances are inseparable from ritual. A performance is presented once. This immerses it in the larger context of life, and undermines the tendency to view art as an object separate from both time and life. The performance has its designated time yet connects participants to the nonlinear "dreamtime" of shamanic culture.

By keeping a performance as simple as possible, artists increase their sensitivity to the environment, the group energy, and the dreamtime. I often introduce performance to a studio group by inviting participants to leave their positions in the circle and move into the center of the group for at least sixty seconds while they practice presenting themselves as images. This elementary change in position, together with the absence of talking, generates a transformative sensitivity to bodily communication. Presence is heightened through silence, and there is an immediate sense of the group's focused energy and the animation of the physical space.

Complex performances distract the mind and insulate the artist. Simplicity enables the performance to become a meditation in which the actor establishes communion with inner movements, the audience, and the space. Like the inner speech of dialogue, action expresses a psychic purpose that flows from sincere and immediate feelings. In discouraging "overacting" Stanislavski said, "never allow yourself externally to portray anything that you have not inwardly experienced and which is not even interesting to you" (1972, p. 28).

Our performance art relates to images that have emerged from paintings and helps the actor to establish bonds to feelings and images that have been "inwardly experienced." The performance offers both an opportunity to reenter the feeling of the experience and to travel to yet another place.

The most familiar actions are transformed when we enter the imagination of the performance. For example, one of our studio participants made a series of paintings of a little man who appeared in a dream. One of his legs was shorter than the other, and he wore a large black hat. The artist was a professional fashion model familiar with walking across a stage before an audience. In her performance she appeared as the dream figure wearing a hat and one high-heeled shoe to create the effect of the short leg. She walked slowly and decisively across the stage, making penetrating eye contact with the audience while the sound of her Ahab-like gait filled the room. The uncomplicated rhythm of the shorter leg thumping down on the floor carried the image of the little man to yet another place in her feelings and in those of the group. He was present in her body. The imaginal figure and the artist were paired in a performance confirming the evocativeness of simplicity.

Performers describe how the enactment "moves something." When they play the image in the painting, it is experienced in another way, and they describe how it is the engagement of the body that deepens the work. Fear before the performance is accepted as "aliveness," which moves the participants "beyond the limits of habit." A performer said, "There is energy behind the fear, and my anxiety brings concentration, presence. The performance is pure presence. I do not think about other things." Another artist described how "the performance draws on energies not accessible by other means. I am different before, during and after." And the audience is essential: "I could not do it looking at the wall. The faces gave me energy."

Dreaming

ALTHOUGH PAINTINGS ARE frequently made in response to dreams, dreams can themselves interpret art with insights that the conscious mind cannot approach. In this way dream experience joins performance, dialogue, and meditation in contributing to the exegesis of a picture. Dreams speak through visual imagery, environments, movements, and feelings as well as words. The following reflections demonstrate the direct and purposeful way in which they contribute to our creative interaction.

In a retreat for art therapists, a woman made a huge painting, at least six feet long, of a barely visible form in black on a dark blue surface. It was her first picture in our residential weekend. She used a great deal of water while painting it, so the image was wet throughout the painting process. When the group reflected on the painting, the artist focused on the dark colors and the relatively formless composition, and she spoke of how she had never painted anything like it before. Her responses were to the sensuous and dark aspects of the image.

The next morning she told the group she dreamt *she was swimming under a boat in deep water, and she looked up to see the dark form of the boat.* She described a sense of danger and excitement and how she swam under boats as a child. She related these feelings to going "underneath" and taking risks during the retreat. The image of the painting was interpreted in a dream that came in response to the painting.

The notion that every part of a dream or painting is a part of oneself, as gestalt therapy asserts, results in the loss of the daimonic world. In this dream for example, the water, the boat, and the swimmer would all be incorporated into the dreamer's ego—the water is an expression of the dreamer's libido, the boat is her life on the surface, the absence of other people expresses her isolation, and so forth—and would lose their autonomy as psychic images. We avoid this "egoism" by simply regarding dream images as figures that appear within the self. In this

128

way we recognize their intimate relationship to us while protecting them from assimilation. By insisting that we relate to images as participants in a mutual interaction, we further their ability to function as psychic agents.

In questioning the idea that psychic images are "parts" of the person through whom they emerge, I do not want to be trapped in dualistic thought. If I say that dream images are not parts of the dreamer, it is difficult to avoid the argument that they are parts, and neither position is capable of positive proof. One of my graduate students approached the situation as a paradox, perceiving the figures in her paintings as parts of herself and wholly other. And why not reverse the context and consider the possibility that we are part of the dream. The novelist Milan Kundera (1991) says that a person's gestures are not individual creations since we cannot make gestures that are completely our own: "it is gestures that use us as their instruments, as their bearers and incarnations."

It is the attitude toward the dream and the artistic image that influences our practice. For example, viewing images as intimate relations reframes the discussion. The notion of "parts" ties us to sums, divisions, physical organization, and self-referential psychology, a perspective that does not correspond to the invisible psychic image. The physical existence of a painting contradicts the idea that it is part of the painter. Our sense of the image as a partner, rather than a part, operates within the frame of relationships. Seeing the image as a part of the self is essentially an expression of a desire for intimate relationship—but being a part takes away its autonomy.

Attitudes determine practice. An emphasis on establishing relationships with psychic images encourages us to entertain them and get to know them better. For example, one-sided reduction of the image to the person's past, even to events of the previous day, can be a flight from the present and the cultivation of the new life that images bring. In our work, history and memory are welcomed as participants in the present interaction.

The woman in my studio received the water, the depths, the presence of the boat, and the purpose of the swimmer. The dream and painting were "related" to her past experiences and influenced by them, but, as Nietzsche said, we are redeemed from the prisons of the past by *creating*. Zarathustra declares, "Break up, break up, ye discerning ones, the old tables!" (1917, p. 207), and he encourages love of our *"children's land."* Every painting and dream is a new birth in which the procreating imagination lives and sustains its generative force.

The practice of reducing dreams to experiences in daily life has generated an equally one-sided practice of regarding them as divine emanations uncontaminated by mundane affairs. This is another instance of needless opposition. Both aspects depend upon one another—divine and mundane, dream and daily life, the gesture and the person who makes it.

Dreams and paintings involve a nonlinear *convergence* of forces—psychic and material, personal and impersonal—which interact to create an event. This perspective on dreams can be related to Corbin's assertion that angels and humans cannot exist without one another.

> Not only does the human being depend upon his Angel, his *Dator formarum*, for all the acts of knowledge that metamorphose him; but reciprocally too, the Angel has need of him to accomplish his own elevation. . . . Tobias and the Angel are here involved in the fate of one and the same pilgrimage. (1988, p. 380)

In order to achieve this partnership, we have to welcome dreams and discover that they never come to harm us. They may startle, puzzle, disgust, and even terrify us, but these provocations are *always* expressions of psyche's wisdom and purpose. For example, guilt and shame about sensual delights experienced in a dream may help us to see that the relationship between the psyche and the body is out of sync.

Strong and troubling communications are often necessary to stir dreamers from anesthetized consciousness. *The Ninja who covers the sleeping woman's head with a net* comes to help her experience her body. *The murderous man with a knife* appears to help another woman cut through and "kill" destructive patterns. *The guillotine in an elegant white Congregational church which is going to kill three young witches* shocks the dreamer into seeing the harm that people can do to one another in groups, even if their purpose is spiritual, and the dream helps him see his anger and get out of his "nice guy" persona when someone strikes viciously. *Hoodlums chase the person*, who awakes in panic and later feels that they are trying to get her attention and acceptance. *The man who kills the wounded wolf to protect his friend* realizes that the wound is the opening to his vulnerability; he can abandon his heroic mode to befriend his wounded soul, his mistreated animal, who is driven to viciousness.

The dream is not to be interpreted literally, and we assist the *agents provocateurs* in eluding the snares of literalism. The literal reading of the dream may limit interpretive meditation. Something that is repugnant in waking life may serve the symbolic purpose of the dream. Yet I do not want to say that dreams never speak literally. Their communications are multifaceted and often include shockingly direct expressions. Even common language can express varied meanings. Owen Barfield has shown how the lexical meaning of a word, phrase, or sentence is expanded by the "speaker's meaning." He says, "The use of metaphor always operates to *expand* meaning" (1967, p. 64). The meaning of a word also changes over the course of history. If these variations characterize our conscious use of language, we can see how unlikely it is to assume that the unconscious and nonlinear expressions of dreams can be reduced to a single and exact meaning. Dreams, like metaphors, expand meaning.

Dreams are vital participants in our art therapy studios. Their emanation closely parallels the making of artistic images, and we respond to dreams in much the same way that we engage paintings. The making of artistic images can be likened to a waking dream. By sharing dreams we immerse our studio in the irradiations of psyche and invoke its manifestations. My meditations on dreams spiritualize my waking life, and there is no doubt that the raw material of what I do each day, the insignificant, subtle, and unwatched experiences, provide the subject matter for psyche's nocturnal art.

A man in a Swiss art therapy retreat was unfamiliar with painting. During our first day he painted conceptual and carefully planned designs, in contrast to the expressive and sweeping gestures that the people around him were making. That night he dreamt *he was making broad and spontaneous Japanese brushstrokes in black ink.* The next day he painted in this style and became the instrument of the dream gesture.

A woman in the same studio was making eight-by-six-foot paintings. She was a tall person, over six feet. With the group she discussed how she feels that she takes too much space and experiences conflicts with others in relation to this. In an evening performance she rolled up one of her large paintings, placed a red rose on it, carried it in a slow procession accompanied by sacred music, placed the painting on an elevated surface, and knelt before it. That night she dreamt that *a large ship stops in the middle of a village to board passengers. It moves deeply through the earth without effort and not subject to the control of a person. As the ship passes, the ground returns to its previous condition.*

These examples show how dreams relate to the daily life of the dreamer. They are themselves art works, soul's dramatizations that help, guide, and extend consciousness. The woman who feels too big, who is accused of taking too much space, and who just walked in a procession, dreams of a large ship that moves gracefully through the earth. It is too simplistic and literal to say that the ship is an image of herself. We lose the magic of the ship by incorporating it into the dreamer. In responding to this dream we marveled at the way psyche amplified the actions of the day, sympathized with them, and transformed them into fascinating forms that reframed the situation within a silent drama of imagery.

Before beginning to lead a small workshop in California, a man from the East dreamt that *he is doing a large session with fifty people, and after a few minutes everybody starts to walk away. The dream ego feels terrible and tells another man that he is angry. The man smiles at him*. The dream put the dreamer into contact with his insecurity and fears of failure. It overwhelmed his self-confidence and defenses and offered an infusion of humility. In reflecting on the dream he began to identify with the man who was smiling at the angry and worrisome person who is the dream ego. "Don't try so hard," he says to ego. "Don't take it so seriously."

During the same night before he began the group, the man dreamt that *the lawn at home is a foot high the day after he cut it*. At first he felt disturbed because the lawn was "out of control," and then he shifted to an aesthetic appreciation of the long grass. As he meditated on the dream he felt its fertility. It was telling him that he cannot control the verdant growth of soul. In both of these dreams the interpretive act involved a shift from the anxious and victimized dream ego, with whom we instinctively associate ourselves, to another aspect of the dream.

Dreams frequently arrive like angels who help the person who tries too hard. *Large, bright bunches of orange carrots grow in fertile soil right behind the dreamer's house*. Potency involves opening to what comes naturally and spontaneously. The dream tells the person that excessive effort leads to labyrinths.

The dream I remember most vividly over the past year left this message gracefully on my doorstep. I had been at a compulsory faculty day where the guest speaker was a young man who struck me as overly enthusiastic about himself. His frantic style of speaking and driving home his points gave me a feeling that he was struggling against himself. I could see my shadow in him. That night *Phil Karpinski, a cool and fluid friend from high school, looks at me after I gave a lecture and says, "You've calmed down."*

Dreams frequently appear to help me relax in my creative work. I dreamt that *I am with my maternal grandfather behind a house. I am hammering a post into the ground* [I could have simply dug a hole]. *It is a stand for a mailbox, and the piece of wood is not solidly in the ground. I feel that the mail should probably go in the front door. Why should the mailman have to go the extra distance to the back of the house?*

The dream tells me to take it easy. My grandfather was skilled in the use of tools, and it was not his style to pound away at something. He is standing silently next to me as I hammer at the post, and I can hear his thoughts saying, "Don't force it." He is the *agathos daimon* (good daimon) who says, "Don't force the communication. It will happen naturally, in its time. Don't worry about the mailman and whether or not he will deliver the letters and where they 'should' go."

Dreams not only interpret life, but they contribute to it. I frequently observe how rites of passage that are overlooked in the day world take place in dreams. At the time I was leaving my job as a dean, I dreamt that I *am cleaning out a large office and placing piles of public relations materials in another room. I am removing crystal glasses from a bottom shelf when a colleague, someone from the early and more adventurous years of my administrative work who has long since left the college, appears and says, "You're not going to clean out the crystal!"* She was a guide telling me not to throw out the precious "family" glass together with all of the impersonal papers. The glass embodied the treasures of the past, memories not to be discarded.

Aesthetic or sensual experiences of daily life can be carried into extraordinary dimensions by dreams. On a fall evening after raking leaves, I lay on the lawn in the dark with my infant daughter and our massive black Labrador retriever, Maximus. He was showing affection by nipping at my neck under the chin. The sky was clear and full of stars, and the waves from the nearby ocean were crashing. That night I dreamt that *I am on a fishing boat with my wife and four children. I see a school of black whales, shut off the engine, and go to sit on the bow, fearful but fascinated. The boat drifts and begins to move at a high speed in a current that enables us to move alongside the whales, which are everywhere. I put my feet over the sides of the bow, hanging them there and trusting. The huge black whales lift their heads, looking like Maximus—Moby dogs. The motion stops and the sea is calm. I speak to my wife.*

In a contemporary and "living" dream life, the artifacts of the present become shamanic tools, which are not restricted to rattles, drums, horses, feathers, and other classical objects. The presence of contemporary artifacts in dreams is an opening to the discovery of divinities in our homes, streets, work places, the devis and devas who flourish in our shopping malls. The *instinctus divinus* is strongest in the most unlikely and therefore most unconscious places. Dreams thus infuse the day world with the divine.

A woman in a studio group described a dream in which the mundane was infused with a psychic vitality. In the dream *she is with her studio companions in her ex-husband's kitchen, looking through cabinets and labeled files. She feels close to his new wife, who looks out the window at the view of a river. He had moved the river to the house, and the new wife says, "He'll do anything I want." The dreamer goes up on the roof of the house where there is an illuminated football field and then she goes down levels of stairs through a sports bar, vaults, and small doors, tight spaces full of wires, pipes, and gauges and progressively lower ceilings, tunnels with an occasional light bulb, a barking dog jumping through chicken wire, a sale in a store with no prices listed, a nude man with unrecognizable words tattooed on his buttocks, armed guards in sequined dresses taking a woman through a barred gate, with everything getting smaller.*

After listening to this dream I felt a contagious animation and drama in relation to the commonplace. Although the dream takes us down through successive levels, the feeling of depth does not "develop." Every moment is as significant as the one before. Scenes constantly dissolve into one another. The ego figure is diminishing at the end and is being led through an underworld gate.

The student saw numerous relations between the dream and her life. For example, the principle of "substitution" is demonstrated here. The dreamer just completed an exciting course with a male teacher, which is analogous to the new wife's delight about the abilities of her husband. As a result of her participation in the training, the student's world was taking on a new vitality, which is expanded by the dream. The tunnels were a continuation of the labyrinthian feeling she had in the city's subways. But the pervasive sense of the dream was the vivification of the ordinary: kitchens, cabinets, football fields, lights, chicken wire, light bulbs, sequined dresses, stores, steps, tiles, wires, gauges, pipes, and miracles performed outside the kitchen window.

In another studio one of the artists had just bought a new sports car that evoked "dream cars" in other participants. One woman dreamt that *she is driving her father's car, an old Volkswagen Beetle with graffiti carved into it*. She thus continued the painting process of the studio in the dream, bringing it home to her family. Another woman, who was driven around during the week in the new sports car, dreamt that *she is painting its windows affectionately*. The aesthetically pleasing car of the day world and the painting we were doing in the studio were fused in both dreams.

The dream helper, or *agathos daimon*, often appears in unlikely and bizarre forms or disguises. For example, *I am showing George Bush how to buy elegant glassware for his wife, Barbara, who is delighted by the gift*. There was a sense in the dream that I was supporting the expression of Mr. Bush's feminine sensibility.

This dream figure of George Bush is an autonomous character, distinct from the literal person. As a daimon he remains intact, and he is experienced for what he is. The mask of George Bush does not necessarily conceal another identity or person. If we accept the dream figure as he is, we become more involved with his psychic function as manifested within the dream and less concerned with trying to figure out who he "represents" within my personal life. The dream figure is a personal acquaintance in his own right.

If I apply the dream to my life, there is an attentive figure within myself who helps the busy man of the world to care for the person with whom he shares daily life.

As mentioned earlier, dreams will often speak directly and without veils. A young man departing from strict observance of family traditions in religion and politics dreamt that *he is sitting in the back of a Gothic cathedral at the funeral of his uncle, the patriarch of the family, and his relatives are in the front with many empty pews between them. As they file out, they glance at him, and he looks to his side, and Lenin is standing next to him*.

The dream not only conveyed separation from family traditions but ritualized the passage within the context of a funeral. The separation was not an aggressive act of rejection but a loss issuing from the process of conscience.

This life-affirming response to the dream as a rite of passage contrasts to the dreamer's first reaction, which evoked feelings of alienation and guilt about breaking family religious traditions. Since the dream embodies feelings of mystery and isolation within a fantastic space, the dreamer may actually have been entering, rather than leaving, the inner sanctum of psyche. He was losing the doctrine and gaining the mystery. The entire experience is an emanation of the Gothic cathedral of imagination.

In addition to interpreting and expanding paintings, dreams have furthered my experience of performance art. In a recent studio that I ran in Switzerland, two men in our group composed largely of women gave an evening performance focused on male interactions and intimacies. They went through a series of awkward attempts to embrace and hold each other. While hugging, one of the men stuck out his behind in order to keep his genital area as far as possible from the other man's. They tied themselves together, back to back, did an athletic dance as a four-legged creature, and ended the piece by holding each other.

In my dream that night *I am driving my father's 1951 Chevy up Avon Hill in Cambridge to my college office. The car is having engine trouble that seems chronic, and one of the front tires is falling apart. The dream shifts to a crowded group of men in a high school lobby. A group of my male college friends are standing together, and I turn and see that my sixteen-year-old son is next to me, and I begin to introduce him with a sense of pride.*

The dream reflects on my history with men, beginning with my father and ending with my son. When I was a boy and the Chevy was getting older, my father said he should save it for me. The chronic ailment of the car is a wound. The wheels of the dream car are falling apart and the engine is dying. My mother now has a degenerative disease and my father is under great stress, yet this crisis is tying us together like the men in the performance.

I was teaching a course in Switzerland, and the appearance of my Cambridge office, my college friends, and my son (who was then applying to colleges) are expressions of the school archetype weaving itself into the dream. The "crowded" group of men in the school lobby corresponded to the feeling I had while watching the men tightly tied together in their performance. The crowding puts me right up against my attitudes toward men.

Someone might say, "You have just reduced every aspect of that dream to your personal life and your past. You contradict what you have said about the autonomous life of the dream."

Contradiction is an essential part of psyche's communications, which do not follow reason's logic. Although I may contradict what I do or say, I do not think that I have reduced the dream to myself. I have felt "connections" between the dream and my life. This sense of linkage and relationship is different from reduction. Dreams use the material of my life and memory to make themselves visible. As I meditate on the dream, I experience the figures as imaginal realities who relate to my life but exist simultaneously in the world of the dream. They were aroused by the performance by the two men, and they depend upon my life in the day world for their activation and formation.

It is the nature of the dream to present untamable experiences beyond the controlled reflections of reason. Labyrinthian dreams take the dreamer into psyche's confusing subways, highways, and impossible passageways. The woman who is trying too hard to figure something out dreams about *a telephone answering machine that talks and records at the same time, while she enjoys flying over the city on a toilet.*

Experience with dreams that recur throughout a lifetime has shown me that we are not always ready to greet the dream and engage it with depth. Psyche's speech in dreams and artistic images is often ahead of us because we are not yet living fully in the present. Recurring dreams indicate how patient and faithful daimones are. They keep coming back until we are ready to receive to them. This readiness involves the recognition of the subtle connections between waking and dream life. Like a Stanislavski Method actor, the person who sees these relationships is one who "remembers."

Subtle and barely conscious experiences in the day world are frequently transformed into the nocturnal drama of dreaming. During the day the dreamer steps into a puddle while getting out of a car and at night dreams of water. While flying in an airplane, an artist in blue jeans glances at a magazine article about a distinguished corporate executive and looks at photos of him in his elegant clothes, and that night he dreams that *he is feeling uncomfortable and poorly dressed while a group of people look at him.*

When the war in the Persian Gulf began in January 1991, a middle-aged man who works as an art therapist caught a glimpse of the French president, François Mitterrand, on television. In his dream that night *his parents, meeting in Paris during World War II, are walking in front of the Louvre. The dreamer's father is in his uniform. The father's brother, a Maryknoll priest, is with them, and the three walk arm in arm.*

As the dreamer reflected on the dream, the words *war baby* came to him, and he realized that his own existence issued from war. He imagined his mother carrying him in her womb in the dream, which includes his familiar and guiding spirits: his parents; the masculine and feminine; an institution for the visual arts; religion; a third force that joins arms with the masculine and the feminine; and a great city of the soul, a place where culture is nourished. His uncle was the oldest of eight, and the dreamer is the oldest of eight. The uncle was a priest, and the dreamer's work is committed to the sacred qualities of art.

I would like to continue reflecting on how dreams interpret art by dialoguing with a dream that relates to a picture that I made in one of my studio groups (see illustration). In the studio where I made this horselike animal, I was busy working with other people and took only a brief time during the weekend for my art. I tried to make a few fast

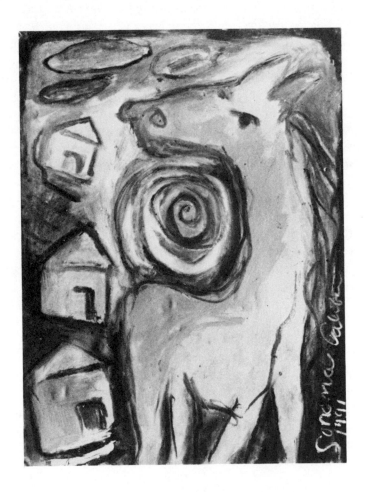

pictures but nothing emerged, so I turned to one of my familiar animals. It faithfully appeared, together with the small buildings or meditation houses that I describe in detail in the next section of this book.

A colleague who was worried about her pattern of painting the same themes over and over again said to me with a smile, "I notice that you do the same thing."

"They are my familiars, my animals," I replied to her. "They bring something different everytime I engage them. They change themselves. I don't have to worry about taking all of the responsibility for making changes. When the ego lets go of the need to make something happen, and when it is ready to listen, the animals will speak and refresh us."

This animal has an elongated neck and a large head. It looks proud, defiant. All of these characteristics are analogous to myself. But this is a creature from another world. Maybe the animal is a psychic cousin. It seems intrigued by the three small buildings. I made the picture quickly, and in place of a tail I introduced the spiral, another of my familiars that often presents itself in a novel way.

The three red clouds are also familiars that appear over and over again. Yet in this picture everything looks fresh, as though I am making all of these forms and figures for the first time. The crowding is unusual. It stirs up the atmosphere and furthers the sense of the picture's individual presence. The animal does not lose composure as a result of everything being so close and stimulating. Its primal instincts and focused senses are intact. I experience the animal as a reliable companion who is comfortable with strong emotions.

In a dream two nights after making the horse and bringing it home from the studio, *I am sitting next to a priest while he performs a ritual for a group. I am gently rubbing an orblike shape under a cloth. It turns out to be the hindquarters of a bronze animal that is a cross between a dog and a horse. The priest reaches over to touch my hand. His touch draws my attention to the unconscious act of rubbing the animal icon.*

The presence of the priest and his ritual suggest a sacred relationship to the animal. The small buildings in my picture have a bronze color, and the animal has taken on their small and solid form in the dream. The rubbing of the hindquarters of the animal is a private act that is simultaneous with the group ritual. The cloth is the veil between worlds. Touch is my mode of entry. There is no thought or reflecting mind in my rubbing, just unthinking sensation and movement.

A Freudian friend says, "Enough talk about daimones and imaginal companions. They are your fantasized defenses against your instinctual desires. This dream is about masturbation and that part of yourself that says 'Don't do it.' You are playing with yourself in front of other people, so don't try to make it more than it is. The priest is the superego figure who tells you to stop by reaching over to touch your hand."

I appreciate this reminder of instinctual basics, which can be overlooked in spiritual meditations. Spiritualizing can become a colorless and restrictive habit. The dream does analogize to masturbation; the animal has phallic characteristics, and I made the picture in the studio in response to a desire for sensuous expression. Comparison to the body's biological functions expands the scope of the dream. They are all aspects of the twists and turns, the constant emanation of psychic life and the playing around that we do. But be wary of locking onto the certainty that the dream means one thing, such as the need for castigation by authoritarian superego figures. Although this Freudian interpreter reverses the format and suggests that guilt is itself the problem, his tone keeps us in the confessional. I muse upon each interpretive perspective as an emanation rather than as the crux to which the dream is definitively reduced. The authoritarian interpreter lives within the perspective of authority and suggests that there is a specific confession to be made. Confession is one of many possibilities that continuously issue from the dream.

If I shift my identification to the priest, the dream is radically transformed. As the leader of the ritual, his function compares with my role in the studio session. Like him, I was responsible for containing the group's actions and providing a sanctuary. My private rubbing of the hindquarters of the animal can be likened to the conflict I felt in the studio about personal expression when I was responsible for the group process. I tried to make this painting discreetly, off to the side of the group, while also attending to what was happening around me. The cloth over the animal in the dream relates to the way in which I did not want my expression to interfere with the group process.

The dream priest speaks: "You were caught at first by your stereotypic image of me as an authoritarian figure, someone who performs conventional rituals with little relationship to your soul and instinctual life. You have to get beyond these habitual notions to empathize with my psychic functions. This connection to authority is from your past, and I exist in the present."

The man who is rubbing the animal says to the priest, "I am feeling different toward you now that you have spoken. I see how I labeled you 'priest,' 'authority,' 'convention.' I realize that we sit close to one another, and the other people in the group are without specific identity. I see four entities in the dream: you, me, the group, and the animal. Perhaps the cloth is a figure too. That makes five of us. The dreamer might consider how these characters interact within him and articulate different aspects of his psychic life. This animal that I am rubbing has no face or upper body that I can see, just hindquarters, lower regions that I touch unconsciously during the ritual. The animal is covered libido."

The animal being rubbed says, "But remember, I am an icon. I am part of the ritual. I bring the instinctual life, the veiled depths in every group. The cloth covering keeps my mystery intact. Libido is only one of my possibilities."

The priest has something else to say, "I did not reach over and touch your hand to tell you to stop rubbing. Do you see the trips that get laid on me because of my role? I was acknowledging what you were doing, and I was 'touched' by the way it contributed to our ritual."

Dialogue between the figures has completely transformed my experience of the dream. I needed their help to get beyond the evaluations of habitual ego theory, that is, that I was doing something wrong, that the private and the social cannot coexist, that the priest is an authority with whom I am in opposition.

The cloth wants to contribute: "We supposedly 'inanimate' objects have to assert our personhood and let you know that we are here. My place in this dream is covering, polishing, and just being rubbed. I am an artifact, and I am totally committed to my role. If you can enter my perspective, you will stop moralizing. You will see that everything has its place and purpose. I am what I do, and that is all that matters. I do not have these confusing thoughts about what I should and should not do. Yet I feel and I play my part sensitively. I cannot be anything else right now."

The dream speaks to the picture: "I continue the life that you generated. I feel related to you but completely different. I am not trying to dramatize the life that you are living, but your textures, forms, and feelings stimulate yet another round of creation through me. The conflicts that your maker had while creating you, his crowded feeling, his lack of space and time, the pressure of his desire and effort, his need to create vital imagery—they are all present abundantly within you, and their life continues to flow through me in a different way. I do not feel an excess in you that passes into me. You completely contain the emotion of your moment in your specific way. There is no overflow, just vitality that influences my appearance. As I look at you now, I see how the smooth hindquarters of my animal relate to you. I also see how the movement of the spiral above your back, along your neck, and below your head can be likened to the circular rubbing motion of my cloth. I am struck by your stature and composure within the crowded atmosphere. The animal instincts of your presence, your colors, textures, and movements, are celebrated in this picture, and they continue to live through me."

The picture replies: "We pass life to one another."

Part Three

DEMONSTRATION

Image Dialogues

IMAGE DIALOGUE IS a mode of the creative process that follows picture making and creates yet another series of expressions. This therapy of the imagination was anticipated by Jung, who introduced all of the creative arts therapies to psychotherapy through his practice of *active imagination,* an inner drama involving the full spectrum of artistic expressions. He described active imagination as "a sequence of fantasies produced by deliberate concentration" on a particular image (Jung, 1969, p. 49). The person watches psyche move and change during the meditation on the image. Images "contain fantasies which 'want' to become conscious," and for Jung "image and meaning are identical." He described inner dialogue as "a touchstone for outer objectivity" (1969, p. 89), intended to further expression of "the unconscious."

My use of dialogue has emerged from a desire to deepen psychological engagement with images and amplify the spectrum of expression. Although it is not possible to show the action of drawing and painting on these pages, my concentration on recent images will, I hope, take us close to the formative movements. The sequence of pictures here does not always correspond to the original series but is consistent with the way imaginal reality rearranges experience according to its intent. I will often introduce a picture by offering a narrative account of how it was created. Although this introduction is generally useful, linear descriptions are at best preliminary to imaginal inquiry. Insight and intimate feelings appear through dialogue and when instinct says to me, "You explain too much." In spite of my incessant admonishing remarks about explanation, I am repeatedly caught in its traps.

The meditations presented here record how drawings and paintings were engaged during a particular moment in time. When walking past these paintings today, different feelings are aroused. This is the nature

of art interpretation that generates new possibilities with each meeting. I realize that talking will sometimes defend against visual experience, and, as Rudolf Arnheim says, verbal expression can be "inferior"
to the language of the image. Dialogue complements "looking,"
which will always be the fundamental response to visual art.

I begin these dialogues by engaging my most recent series of pictures, five oil pastels made while I was leading an art therapy studio in
Switzerland. The studio coincided with the beginning of the Persian
Gulf war. We gathered in a retreat setting in the Swiss mountains
overlooking Lake Constance, and the sanctuary was penetrated by the
war, which influenced pictures, performances, dreams, and group
interactions.

Not only is the individual imagery of the ordinary psyche influenced
by the world, but perhaps the obscure and often unconscious musings
of individual souls also send something back to the larger context. We
typically feel powerless with reference to geopolitical processes that
haunt our interior lives. The medicine of art gives us the opportunity
to take private and small actions which send out ripples of consciousness affecting others. Art replaces apathy and hopelessness with focused action within the realm of the individual imagination and its
visions of the world.

These first dialogues are concerned with compassion for those on all
sides who suffer from violence. I reflect on the war imaginally and
approach it as a global outbreak of aggression that triggers personal
memories, fears, and desires. Following this first series, the pictures
and dialogues move inward. The pathologies and conflicts of the external environment act as openings to the interior.

Figure 1 expresses a sense of homage to the landscape and to nature,
and fantasies about ancient Babylon. It was made just before the
fighting began. The earth is green. The dogs are alert, and they smell a
change in the weather, a coming storm. The figures look vulnerable in
the open space. They are easy targets.

These two are religious men. The one on the ground could be
bowing in prayer, or he might be distraught or exhausted. He is close
to the earth, to the lower regions of the picture, to instinct. The
standing figure watches over the other man without interfering. He is
a silent witness who stands between his companion and the animals.
There is a neutrality and plainness in their clothing, especially the gray
trousers. The picture's emotions seem to shift between devotion, sadness, and heightened sensation.

The dogs are watching over the men.

Nobody wants to speak. They are enveloped by the silence of the vast space.

The small building is odd, mysterious. It has something to say:

"What am I doing here in this open space? I feel a bond to those two men. I have the lavender color of their shirts in me, and we are together as a group of three in this section of the picture. My lavender and pastel colors suggest mystical bliss. I am also between the men and the distant city. But I am not a house in which people live or work, and I am not a temple or a place where rituals are performed. I am a mystery, a place of the imagination.

"I am settled into the space between the two men and my door is open to them, but they are unable to come inside right now. I wonder if the man on the ground knows that I am here? Is his heart open or closed? I don't know what I can do for him. I will stay here with my

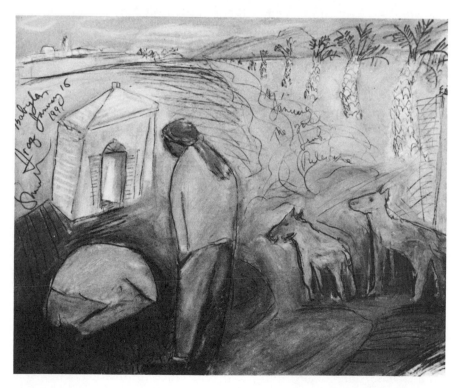

Fig. 1

door open, and maybe he will feel that he is not alone. Why am I always trying to help? He is probably fine without me. I cannot save these men from the things that threaten them. I feel as though I am floating and disconnected from their daily lives. But I am always here waiting, and I will be ready if they need me.

"From the outside I appear to be a small cubicle, but I open into expansive interior spaces. My inner colors are green, and when you pass through the door you will see that there are no walls or ceilings. People enter me through imagination. My physical structure is only intended as a suggestion, a charm, for meditation. I take on this visible form in order to offer a bridge to other realms. I am a passageway, the shaman's doorway."

Before the small building spoke, it was an enigma, just an unusual form that found its way into my picture. A shift has taken place as a result of its speech.

I am involved with a fertile and "green" imaginative process that was not present before. I was feeling stuck, superficial, and restricted. Nothing was happening. I knew that I needed some help, and I decided to trust the artistic process and see what it delivered. The theme of how the struggle for survival makes it difficult or impossible to go to places of prayer and reflection came through the dialogue. I did not think of that angle before. All of us in the Swiss art therapy studio were similarly caught between our purpose for gathering in a retreat setting and our preoccupation with the war.

The building has come forward as a figure that takes me into imagination. One of my graduate students in Cambridge had painted a similar form, and I was intrigued by the way it existed somewhere between symbol and architectural structure. If the building were more complex, it would lose its magical quality. The student said that the building she painted was a "tardis," a structure that appeared in the British television series *Dr. Who*. I discovered from my student that the tardis, which was apparently modeled after a London telephone booth, also opens to extended areas. The image flies from psyche to psyche.

Enough anecdotal reflection. The building wants to talk again.

"Don't you see? I am the opening to imaginal dialogue. I have come to help you. Don't just look at those men as Iraqis. They are psychic figures, your familiars. That one on the ground suggests your inability to talk, your inability to look, *your* reluctance to open to new vistas. He is the one who cannot look out at the wonders of the world because then he will have to change. He actively resists. Of course you care about the Middle East, but your usefulness will be lost if you allow yourself to be absorbed by a single point of view. You will be captured by it, as he is, and you will not be able to sympathize with that which opposes you. Psyche is unpredictable, full of surprises."

I respond, "The man on the ground no doubt corresponds to my reluctance to change, my feeling of being stuck. But right now I see him as self-effacing. He bends to honor the earth, the depths of psyche. He is meditating on primal things. I painted him as an Iraqi in sympathy with the common people of that country. He evokes several emotions. I have to be free to continuously restate my relationship to him."

The standing figure is the man of habit. He is heavier, not very anxious, and he wears common working clothes. He is sincere, responsible, and he responds to people when they are in need. He always gets the job done, but he follows the same patterns each day, doing things that are assigned to him.

The dogs are starting to engage my imagination. They are off to the side of the picture, but they are not peripheral. They stand in an area of rich green. The man on the ground is surrounded by the same dark green. Lighter greens are in the distance. The dogs face the men, and the fact that there are two of them suggests that they have a soul connection to the men, perhaps as companions or as instinctual guides. But they are not expressions of the animal qualities of the men or the artist who made the picture. Seeing them in that way reduces them to extensions of human beings. They are independent figures who interact with the humans during daily life and within the imagination.

For the first time I see a relationship between the animals and the building. They face one another from opposite sides of the picture, and the men are between them. For a moment I thought that the small building, the animals, the palm trees, and even the mountains and distant city were surrounding the men and making a sanctuary for them. But that would make these images subservient to the human presence. I am shifting my perspective to see the humans as part of a circular movement that includes all of these elements.

The keen instincts of the dogs enable them to anticipate movements and sense thoughts. They are perspicacious creatures, and they want to speak.

"So you are just beginning to realize that our color is the same green that you see inside the building. It is more difficult for you to imagine life from the perspective of the animal. Why don't you forget about your thoughts for a minute and reflect upon our yellow-green color? This color is the meeting place between the darker greens below us and the yellows above. We domestic animals live between shadows and light, between humans and wildlife.

"You are beginning to pay attention to the doorway you penciled just above us on the edge of the paper. There is an exit sign above the door, an old symbol from pictures you made years ago. We are not interested in leaving. We are present. The palm trees that you frequently put into your pictures are a signature, a link with the past, an expression of your phallic nature. There are so many trees but you keep them in line. They diminish in the distance, and the closest one touches the exit door."

The dogs continue, "We are energies of the present and we point into the picture and toward the mysterious house. We have taken you into imagination and out of the offices. The exit sign always appeared in your paintings of offices and meetings because you wanted to get out. You drew it in here next to us to tell yourself that we were what you were after. We were on the other side of those doorways. We are nature, instinct, the life that opens the doors of imagination. You are beginning to think that the mysterious building may be our house, the residence of psychic figures and mysteries."

The doorway with the exit sign was placed into the picture in response to structural and aesthetic problems, to modify the bland stretch of green to the right of the tree and the area between the tree and the dog. It was that space and the composition of the picture rather than a personal history with doorways that influenced the change. The picture wanted movement and contrasting lines.

When the image of the door arrived, it began to stimulate imagination and take on psychic significance. This is an example of how images in paintings can never be reduced to aspects of the artist's emotional history. The image came into existence in response to a technical problem on the periphery of the picture. The psychic reflections that I am describing take place afterward. They are another phase of the creative process, deepening my experience of the picture and taking it into the realm of psyche. My interaction with the picture is not limited to the resolution of compositional problems. And I have not attempted to say what the doorway "means." I meditate upon its relation to my life and its archetypal significance as an image with a history of its own.

It is true that the doorway with the exit sign is one of my familiars. It is a form that I choose to repeat in my pictures, and it must appeal to my aesthetic and psychic sensibilities. In this respect it becomes a symbol of continuity. But like any other aspect of my past, it does not have a fixed meaning. I re-create my relationship to the doorway whenever it enters the picture. It is almost transparent, and it now strikes me as a door of eternal passages. The same applies to the doorway in the small building. I am forever passing through them, changing, and going nowhere in particular. I feel connected to the man on the ground, to the man who watches over him, to the dogs who also stand by, and to the earth.

The man on the ground is not distraught. I was distraught, and I am attributing this feeling to him.

The picture may not be saying anything about my sadness and mixed feelings about the war. The man is making primal contact with the earth, with the green. He is involved with the inner life, yet fully present in the external world with its light and shadows. He has a witness or guide, animal familiars, the spirit of nature, and a humble temple of the imagination. The city is distant because he is on retreat. The Middle Eastern city is also one of my familiar artistic images.

This is a better beginning for dialoguing with images than I realized when I first looked at the picture. I feel open to expression now and was not earlier. Meditation has helped me to see that this is a picture about beginnings, passages, and travels into vast spaces in the company of familiar figures. I began my dialogues with this picture because it was the first one I did in the Swiss studio from which I just returned. When I began these reflections, the image did not feel particularly significant. Emotional distance and a lack of connection to images frequently characterize the beginning of an art therapy session. I have to take considerable time with an image, meditate on it, return to it over and over again, get to know it as something with an autonomous life whose nature is elusive, and then the analogies and connections to my life begin to present themselves. I move into the expressions and psychic labyrinths that open themselves to me through the image. The paths are manifold and sometimes contradictory. It is important to give the image the freedom to contradict itself. Similarly, I try to let the analogies change and restate themselves.

This extended dialogue suggests a way of interpreting images that has little resemblance to the prepackaged conclusions that are all too often associated with the psychological interpretation of art. Just this evening my five-year-old daughter gave me an example of good art interpretation. She held up a small clay animal that she made and said, "Daddy, it can be anything. Today it's a wildcat."

The bent-over man in my picture has been listening to all of this, and he says, "I am amazed at the way my position here on the ground suggests so many things to you."

Figure 2 is another picture that I made just before the war with Iraq began. I was reflecting on the Tigris and the Euphrates rivers in Babylon. These pictures communicate feelings about the conflict, as contrasted to the repetitious analysis we were hearing on the media. The constant talking and explaining and strategizing felt like defenses against the true nature of the event.

I serve as chairperson of the board of trustees of an Israeli graduate institute that I helped to establish in 1980. I frequently travel to the region, and my closest colleague is an Iraqi Jew. He is a native speaker

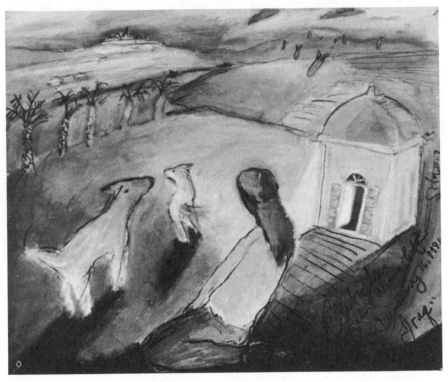

Fig. 2

of Arabic who emigrated to Israel as a young man. Like many of my Israeli friends, he longs for creative cooperation with the Arab world. We imagine the possibility of driving in a car from Tel Aviv to visit Damascus, Beirut, and "someday in Baghdad," his native city. As I describe this relationship, I begin to liken the two men in figure 1 to the two of us. Experience in Israel has deepened my respect for all of the cultures and religions of the region.

When I first reflected on figure 2, I thought that my pleasant landscape, with its reddish-orange jet planes and falling bombs and barely discernible tanks in the distance, was a way of avoiding the unfolding hostilities. I had not drawn jets, tanks, and bombs since I was a child in the 1950s. I saw the picture as an expression of a child's innocent vision.

The religious figure is more relaxed here, and he looks at the dogs and the landscape. Like the figures in the previous picture, his head is covered by a *kaffiyeh*, the red-and-white cloth worn by Iraqi men, bound by the cord known as an *agal*. The small building appears again, and it looks more like a prayer house or a sanctuary in this picture. It was originally sitting on top of a four-sided pyramid of steps, but it looked too lofty and did not fit into the landscape as a whole, so I leveled the steps. It is now on the same plane with the man and the dogs. The light turquoise of the roof suggests a meeting between earth and sky. It evokes Native American culture as well as the turquoise domes of the Muslim world. It is a soothing and healing color. The cool blue inside the building corresponds to the peacefulness of reflection, a place to care for the soul, healing through imagination. The blue water separates the foreground of the picture from the tanks and the distant city, but bombs are falling close to the building. The lavender color is in the building again, with other pastels and a vertical line of bright yellow. The colors in this picture are vivid and distinct. They ask for an interpretive response. There is also lavender in the man's shirt, which connects him to the house, as does his posture. He leans back. His body, the line created by the two dogs, the line of trees, the river, and the horizon, all take the eye up to the airplanes and their orange bombs.

Someone in the studio walked by the picture and said the house looked like a safe place. I realized that in going back to the motifs of my childhood art, I was thinking about the children who would be affected by the war. I imagined myself and my four children as Iraqis.

At the bottom of the picture I wrote, "Charm for the protection of children."

The picture is a meditation on protection and innocence. The military artifacts are overwhelmed by the bright colors. But this is wishful thinking and a denial of what they do. The dogs are pastoral and elegant. They are expressions of innocence, beautiful forms of life that do not choose war or contribute to it in any way.

A voice asks, "Why are you so concerned with protecting Iraqis? What about Israeli children and American soldiers? It sounds like you have taken sides."

Sympathetic imagination transcends the polarization of sides. I made this picture just before "our" bombs began to fall on Iraq. When the missiles were falling in Israel, I was on the telephone with friends, and I visited Tel Aviv during the war. Every life is inviolate. As an ordinary person, I contribute to stopping the spirals of violence by feeling compassion for the other, and especially those who are labeled "evil." Soldiers and politicians do not have to carry all of the responsibility for the archetypal drama of war and changing its expression. Imagination enters the mythology of war without choosing sides. We acknowledge its archetypal purpose and find alternative ways of expressing its destructive energy. I do this through art.

The two dogs are animated. The falling bombs and the beauties of nature are juxtaposed. War breaks out in perfect weather and in a spectacular landscape.

At first the dogs appeared to be playing. Now I see them sniffing the air with apprehension. They know that something is wrong. Their movements could become frenzied. They are ready to speak.

"We cannot trust the world to you humans. What are those thunderous and screeching sounds? Do your prayers bring these noises?"

The man says, "This is all fantasy. It is happening in the distance. I am here in my tranquil place with my dogs, the garden, the river, and the views of the city. It does not concern me."

Let's use Hillman's device of restating the scenario.

When the man looks up from his work in the garden, the dogs are aroused, the tanks arrive, and the bombs begin to fall.

Or from yet another perspective, when the planes arrive and the bombs begin to fall, the dogs are startled and the man falls down on his knees.

The picture is starting to look like a dream, full of contradictory elements. The man is relaxed, and intrigued by the aesthetics of war. I had a similar experience in the Golan Heights during Israel's war in Lebanon. Rockets were going off, and I was struck by the power of the sounds and the beauty of the landscape. In this picture there is a moment of exquisite beauty before the bombs fall. I made the image before the bombing of Iraq started, perhaps hoping that it would not occur. This picture involves a state of being suspended between worlds.

The man says, "War has become entertainment and stimulation. The biggest, longest, and most successful television show in history. Unlike the animals with their instinctual wisdom and grace, we humans need a colossal battle, an outbreak of our most extreme pathology, to awaken ourselves."

The small building is tired of being described with religious images such as prayer houses and sanctuaries.

"I have nothing to do with temples. I am simply a building and I am here together with the other parts of the picture. I have no relationship to the man or the dogs or the landscape other than the fact that we happen to be in the same picture. I do not belong here. I feel out of place. But now that I am here, I am part of the environment together with the others, and I will commit myself to them. It could be otherwise, but it is not. This is the existence that I have been given, and I will live it fully. Each of us just arrived—I, the dogs, the man, the city, the river, the planes, and the bombs. People try to make the different parts fit into a single theme. They always want to organize us into an explanation. I am here and I do not know why, but I will do whatever I can with the situation.

"I have no idea who that man is or where the dogs came from. And I don't know what I am or what I have inside me. You look through the open door and see a rich blue color inside me, a watery blue. Perhaps I open to water and dreams. I am a small building in a vast space. But I contribute to the world by living my life fully in this particular place.

"If you look at my physical qualities, you will see that I have delicate and refined lines, pinkish, fleshy, and light blue colors. I evoke reverie and a sense of interiority. I am the antithesis of war."

The red sky is beginning to look like fire, blood, massive heat, an alchemical burning, but it is all highly controlled. The picture is almost sickeningly pretty, neat and carefully planned. Where is the destruction, the suffering?

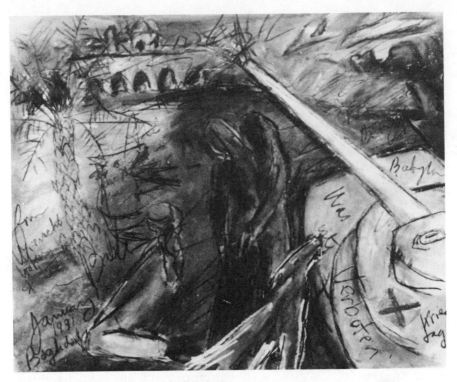

Fig. 3

The spiritual and hopeful yellow and the city of light in the distance are denials of the pain to come. Oh my God, it's the hopeful yellow, the omnipresent yellow ribbons that anger me because they seem designed to channel our response to this war into a prefabricated, Disney-like sentimentality. Although I know the ribbons are deeply meaningful to the families of those involved in the conflict, for me the prospect of war evokes complex personal emotions that cannot be contained by this mass-produced symbol.

The war had begun, and I felt that the previous picture was too controlled, too cerebral, too calm, so I aggressively scribbled the picture shown in figure 3. It is the first one I made after the bombing started. I intentionally drew the kneeling man again in order to change his environment. The open space is gone. This one is crowded, dark, explosive, and closer to the underworld and the smells of war. After working with oil pastels, I took my black pencil and scratched at the picture to increase the turmoil. To embody the violence of war, the motions while painting had to be correspondingly violent. The tank with its cannon came in toward the end of the process because the composition needed something intrusive, large, and penetrating. The picture expresses disarray and does not take sides. War occurs in a city at night where it affects noncombatants. The tank has a bold X insignia on it, and I wrote in broken German, "What is forbidden? War day, January 17, 1991." Two women traveled from Berlin to work in our Swiss studio, one of whom had lived through the Second World War. The conflict in the Persian Gulf was stirring a psychic cauldron of memories.

The dog has turned on the tank. The three people just look and listen. The picture was not aggressive enough, so I made another angry and distorted beast, showing its open mouth, just above the tank on the right side of the picture. It still is not torturous enough. I actually enjoyed working with the dark umber color, with black and gray, and felt how the aesthetic sense is sometimes heightened in moments of danger and terror.

The picture says, "I have been drawn from the vantage point of one who looks and who is outside the violence. The artist is not in the chaos. He is cool, removed, and he sits in his blue temple of imagination in order to sense what it is like here. He reflects and organizes a composition of characters, each of which has its place within the painting. I am a polite picture and I do not assault the viewer. The bombs and the fire are falling in the distance, a safe distance."

The woman on the right with her left arm on the hip of the man says, "Can we fight? Are we capable of it? We are numb. What does this destruction do to us? The American pilot on the television said Baghdad looked like a Fourth of July celebration. Another said the city looked like a Christmas tree. It is eerie how devastation has its aesthetic appeal, its beauty. The sounds and vibrations are extraordinary. The earth shakes. What is our perspective? What does it look like to us? I want to stand here amid the violence and experience it. This is the only thing I can do, experience it, witness it, and I will remember it. Otherwise I am helpless.

"The dog acts without thinking, without ambiguity. It is angered. But soon it will be frightened and it will find shelter. Its instincts know that this open plaza is no place to be. The war will eventually come closer."

I was just considering how I should make another, more grim and aggressive image of the war in order to get closer to its violence and the consciousness of innocent victims. But trying to get "better" at expressing the situation abandons this image.

The man who is kneeling has settled into the situation. He says, "Everything is right here. Relax and settle into your feelings. If you run off to another picture, you will leave what is happening here. Don't force your response. You have been known to overdo it, to try too hard. Aren't you showing an insecurity about your expression in trying to make another image? Maybe this image is upsetting to you."

Although it is necessary to let go of attachments and go on to new creations and situations, I often move too quickly. Action becomes an anesthetic. The positive trait quickly turns into its shadow.

That last line, "Maybe this image is upsetting you," is opening a new wave of feelings about the image. The picture is now upsetting me. The red in the upper right is no longer fire. It is blood in the air, a spray of blood. It evokes memories of the violent and tragic death of my young sister, struck by a speeding car. Last night I came across some lines from Shakespeare's *Romeo and Juliet* that I wrote down when she was killed:

> Death lies on her like an untimely frost
> Upon the sweetest flower of all the field.
>
> . . . .
>
> Death, that hath ta'en her hence to make me wail,
> Ties up my tongue, and will not let me speak.

Reflecting on my picture evoked this upsetting memory from my personal life. This does not mean that the picture can be reduced to that particular memory. They are related but distinct. The psychological interpretation of art has often confused similarity with identity. Artistic images offer resources for considering how different forms of life relate to one another. Psychological reductionism will see my picture of the war in the Persian Gulf as an expression of the traumatic loss of my sister. If we look at the process of interpretation as analogy, then my personal memory is *related* to the picture I draw of the war. Analogy enables images and artists to maintain their autonomy while also interacting with one another and establishing sympathetic connections. "Staying with the image" enables the analogies to appear and take hold.

L'agent provocateur is here again and says, "Why are you going off on this tangent? Haven't you said enough about interpretation problems? You are taking me away from emotion. When you were tempted to make another picture of the devastation to get it right, didn't the kneeling man say, 'If you run off to another picture you will leave what is happening here'? You are doing it again. That's twice!"

I was running away from the emotion surrounding the tragic death of my sister. It "ties up my tongue, and will not let me speak." I did not know what to say, how to respond. All I could do was stop. The identification of the red as blood in the air stunned me. It slipped into the dialogue unexpectedly. When I began to talk again, the intellectual distancing occurred. I unconsciously reacted with, "Let's change the subject."

The wound connects me to the suffering of innocents everywhere. The personal is archetypal.

Five months before Iraq invaded Kuwait, I made a large painting in my studio of a pack of wolflike dogs gathered outside a walled Arabic city. It was very strong and took up a great deal of space, so I thought, "No one is going to want to look at this." I painted the figure of a reclining woman over the animals and left a solitary dog in the picture. I include the painting at a later point in this section (fig. 24). The dogs of war were replaced by a large female figure. That is not interpretation but a description of what I did. The feminine is filling my pictures, and a psychological interpreter will say that I am coming into contact with my feminine. Others will insist, "He is obsessed with women."

I do not know why the woman appears in figure 4 (page 160). I instinctively made her. She comes in response to the bombs and destruction in the previous picture. It is the same pattern of a reclining woman taking the place of threatening animals. This image infuses the feminine into the series. I do not see her as a denial of the violence. She comes in response to it. I am struck by the vitality of the colors, her purple dress, the lavender dogs, the yellow hair and trees, the blue river, the soft grays in the background, the red and white of the Swiss flag. The dog at the left is surrounded by light green-yellow, and the one at the right is enveloped by a rich, deep blue. The dogs take on different functions as a result of the way they are framed in color. The dog in the blue seems to be her protector, who stays in the shadow, whereas the dog in the light may be leading her. Both dogs are turned toward her. The more I look at this picture, the more I am affected by

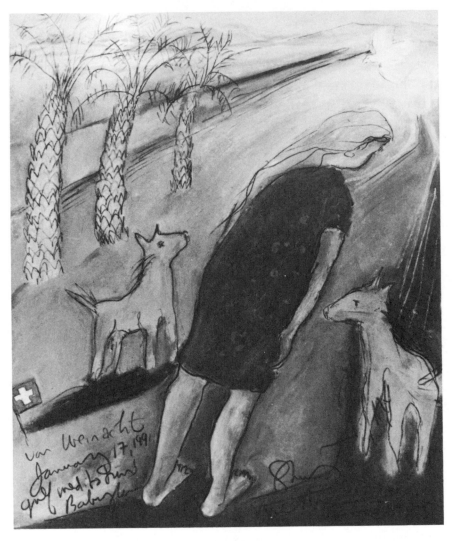

Fig. 4

the colors, especially the passion and feeling of her purple. She is an emotional response to the devastation of the world. The small white bird at the top right connects me to the white in the tiny Swiss flag at the bottom left. Her bare feet are a bond to earth. It is the best antidote I can make to war.

The small building from figures 1 and 2 appears faintly in the distance. I wanted to add something new to the picture, something fertile. The river behind the three palm trees is the same shape as the tank cannon in the previous picture. So it's as if the cannon became a river.

I am not saying that I unconsciously made the cannon into a river. All I can say with certainty is that I see the formal relationship between the two, and I make these connections afterward, through interpretive reflection. The cannon and the river are brought together through my meditations on the images, which does not make the relationship less significant. To insist that the connections were made on an unconscious level during the process of drawing is psychologically and artistically irrelevant. What ultimately matters is the fact that this connection has been made, and it stimulates imagination and curiosity. It opens up new possibilities for viewing the series of pictures. By reflecting on this similarity, we are saying that the pictures are related to one another. Our methods affirm the interrelationship of images within the psyche. But we do not want to force the process of making connections between pictures, because they are also distinct from one another. For example, this picture "interrupts" the movement toward war in the previous images.

The woman needs to speak.

"No, no, no. I can still say no to what is happening around me. I can turn to the greening of this life. I am not helpless. I can create. I can change my small life."

She has the help of the animals. The small white dovelike bird appeared near the end of the river without contemplation on peace symbols. It just flew into the corner of the picture. It is very small and the same ethereal color as the building below it. The bird's wing actually touches the building, whose tiny shape reinforces the relationship to the bird. Everything in the picture converges toward that corner. There is a strong thrusting movement toward a soft, minute, and dreamy objective. The woman leans toward this area, and her head nearly touches the bird and the building.

She reflects on the sanctuary, "The environment of the building is a dream, but I am going to stay with it. I am going to keep it inside me. I will not let it go even though it has grown small and insubstantial. Everyone has access to its creative magic, but it is slipping away. I will not let it disappear. I will keep it in my memory."

The dove says to the artist who made the picture, "You have soft and delicate sensibilities. You are exercising them in this picture, keeping them close to you. The bird of Elysium has not flown away. It exists. The little sanctuary is still there, and you have colors, animal companions, and feminine sensibility. She is walking without shoes, feeling the ground and the morning moisture. Yes, we are still here, soothing colors and images, water, the palm trees, the woman. She turned her back on the war. She threw her shoes at the planes. The animals are comforting her. She will regenerate the earth and the cities. And she will not forget. She will watch over the sanctuary of creation."

The small Swiss flag at the lower left appeared as an afterthought, as a signature of place. I often put flags into pictures that I make in foreign countries to acknowledge the spirits of the place where I am working. I have a feeling of reverence for these flags, and I feel connected to all of them. The Swiss flag looks incongruous in this imaginary scene of the Middle East, but this incongruity may help reveal qualities of the picture that I have not seen.

Nationalism makes no sense here—a Swiss flag with a blond Western woman walking through the psychic environment of the Middle East drawn by an American man—or perhaps it makes perfect sense. The life of imagination opens to all perspectives, to identification with all countries, religions, genders, places, and forms of life—a "multiverse" rather than an "universe," as one of my graduate students said to me. I put the flag into the picture as an afterthought and I am talking about it now as an afterthought and that is how I feel about nationalism. It is an afterthought to the sanctity of life.

The confrontational voice says, "You are a romantic escapist. You flee from the terrors of war with your soft fantasies."

"Romantic escapist"—hostile critics are fond of labels.

The romantic aspect does not deny or avoid the violence. This picture came in response to the war. There is no contradiction within imagination. Soul needs sanctuaries, safe and loving places where life regenerates. A sanctuary can be a very small part of life, a tiny building or space where imagination escapes drudgery and nourishes itself. The ax-grinders, grandiose egos, and apocalyptic moralizers could use a daily spell in small romantic rooms.

The last picture in the Swiss series is shown in figure 5. Every gesture seemed to fall into place, and few parts of the picture were reworked and changed. It takes us closer to the city, and there is interaction among masculine, feminine, and animal aspects. I con-

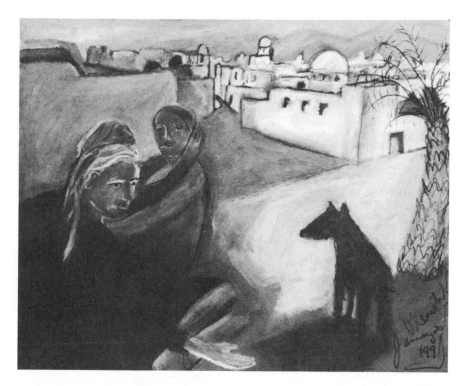

Fig. 5

structed a city amid the war. It is an intimate and gentle scene that once again emerged without planning or prior reflection on a theme.

The woman in the foreground attracts my eye. She is calm and extending an open hand to something that is outside the picture.

"Come and join us," she says. "Sit with us in the shade."

The dog seems to accompany whatever it is that we cannot see.

The man is looking at the woman, and he is supporting her. He does not speak, but his silent thoughts are saying, "You relax me."

The other woman is trying to capture his attention.

"Look at me. Pay attention to me. You are always off with your fantasies. You want what you cannot have. I am here with you. Look at me. I am physical and I am touching you."

The man has nothing to say. He just looks and feels.

The figures and the dog are in earth tones, yellow ocher and burnt sienna. The colors and posture of the human figures connect them to the animal and the ground. There is a dark umber at the backs of the women. They look as though they are closer to the realm of the animal than they are to the world of the city in the distance. They seem to be outside the city, but they might also be in a plaza. Perhaps they are sitting outside their house.

The animal is attentive and curious about what the people are doing. It seems comfortable with them, yet its placement apart from their grouping, and closer to the tree suggests that its role is one of watching over them. It reminds the people of their animal nature and sensory ties to the earth. The reddish brown of the burnt sienna in the animal, the man, and the woman in the foreground is the same color as the rich, sandy soil in Israel. I have always been struck by the contrast in soil colors and textures in different parts of the world. The red earth of the Middle East is so different from New England's dark umber soil. I put umber in the bottom left, behind the woman, perhaps to support her back. I was not consciously applying colors with these thoughts. They emerge as I reflect on the image.

The dog and the palm tree constantly appear in my pictures. Their presence affirms the past. In this image they look relaxed. The palm tree is one of the most animated figures in the picture. Perhaps it can move and speak. It is more active than the seated figures. It fills the right side of the image. It stands there like a guardian with the dog. The tree literally connects the area where the people are sitting to the city. Its branches hover over the small doorway that leads my imagination into the inner sanctum of the city. The warm yellow color of the tree is welcoming.

The tree says, "I have been planted here to serve as a link between worlds. The city is waiting. You can pass into her mysteries when you are ready. She is all of the places that you have seen and have yet to see. She is the architecture of your imagination, a dream labyrinth of new rooms, new vistas, blue skies."

It looks like a holy city combining masculine towers and feminine openings. It is situated at the top of the picture and highlighted with rose colors and light blues, which mediate between white and red, white and blue. This placement and the presence of the mountains give me the impression that it is a city of the spirit, of endless possibilities. The woman in the foreground, by contrast, is a creature of the earth. I begin to see her as the keeper of Nature's secrets.

Now my sense of the other woman is beginning to change. She

looks like the helper of the woman in the foreground, and she soothes the man: "Don't be afraid. We will show you the way. You can leave behind the city of your thoughts, your planning, your conquests, and we will take you into our mysteries."

He looks respectful, contemplative, and immersed in the feminine. They could be involved with Orphic sacraments that meditate on the creative forces of nature. His masculine presence, together with the animal, complements the feminine principles. Yet in this image the primary sense is one of women's mysteries rather than men's.

He is thinking, "I want to live my life in another way, closer to the animals and the earth. I am pleased that these women trust me and include me in their rituals. They are the feminine sensibilities of psyche. It is good to become better acquainted."

The movement in this series toward the feminine and the animal has characterized my art for over two years. Even the upheavals of war cannot keep me away from it. The woman appears out of the conflict. She does not resolve it. She just appears and evokes the mysteries of creation. The man interacts with her.

I keep placing the image shown in figure 6 (page 166) on top of a pile of thirty other pictures that I made over the past few months. I feel relief when I look at it. The movement is appealing. This dreamy flight is not in the previous pictures. The bending motion of the palm tree is repeated in the body of the woman and again in the curves in front of the small building. I am seeing this pattern for the first time.

This is the second version of a man grasping a woman while the two of them are in flight. The first version was an oil painting, and my wife liked the gesture, so I did it again, focusing more on the figures in this one. It does not feel like a sexual picture as I look at it now, and I was not concerned with sexuality when I made it. I am struck by the effort to grasp, to hold, and she cannot be contained. It feels like the effort the artist makes to engage soul, which is forever elusive. It is her nature to be elusive. She may be contacted, but the engagements are fleeting and she is never encapsulated by consciousness. In figure 6 the man clings to the woman with everything he has, and she is so relaxed. His Herculean exertion contrasts to Aphrodite's repose. Both of these aspects are present within the artist's psyche together with the tree, the atmosphere, and that mysterious vaultlike building without windows. The picture gives me a sense of delight because of the way it embodies dreamy tranquillity together with his need to hold her. She illustrates

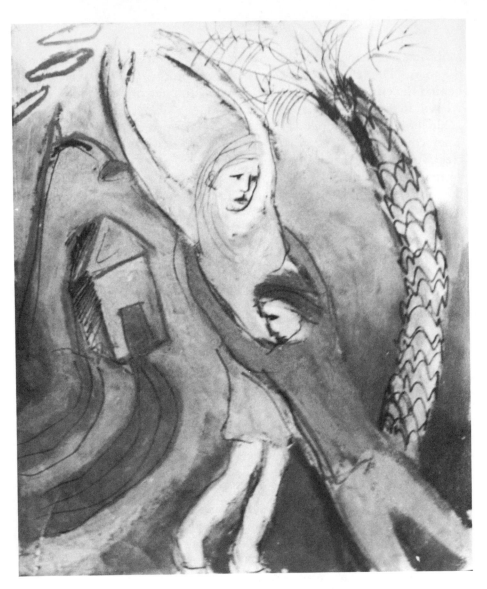

Fig. 6

166

Melville's line in *Moby Dick* about the "ungraspable phantom" of life. I have been obsessed with that phrase for years.

This picture was made a few months before figures 1 through 5, and it is the first response to my student's "tardis." The appearance of the image here can be viewed as a psychic "theft" engineered by Hermes, the guide to the traveling soul. The house can also be imagined as an autonomous image that passes from artist to artist. This simplified version of the house had been emerging gradually as part of a more pervasive effort to simplify architecture in order to experience "primary" forms. My student's image inspired me to make it even simpler. My houses maintain three dimensions, however, whereas the ones in her drawings are flat and two-dimensional.

These secondary, or background, images may be as significant as what appears in the foreground.

I spoke recently to the student about the way the image has been appearing in my pictures. She smiled and said that one of her friends saw the tardis that she was drawing as "home plate" because of its presentation in flat, frontal views. The way in which the sides of the house in my picture are shaded deemphasizes the third dimension, and I am now seeing it as an arrow pointing up. Maybe it has something to do with direction or travel.

This structure does not appear to have anything to do with the normal functions of a house, and it does not seem to contain anything. It stands there as a mystery, and the bright red doorway is wide open. The illuminated red looks like an inner space rather than a closed door.

I would like to shift to what is going on between the man and the woman.

She says to him, "I am not your savior. You are going to have to do it alone. Your obsession with me keeps you unconscious. This relationship is not going to be your salvation. You have to find that on your own. I do not want the responsibility for your salvation. I do not want to be used. As soon as the novelty wears off, you will go looking for something else."

Now a different aspect of the feminine speaks. "I do not want to be restrained by you, controlled by you. You are so needy."

The man reflects on his longing. "I have been without feeling and inspiration for so long. This new desire is thrilling. Everything is alive in the environment. Your inaccessibility is just fine. I do not need to possess you or control you. I just want to feel this desire for you. I keep moving toward you, and you are always out of reach. Even now, as I lunge and appear to hold you, you slip away effortlessly."

Someone suggests that the tree is a phallus and that the man's desire is sexual.

He replies, "So, you think this tree is phallic. Why not! I can open myself to the analogy and imagine the tree as an image of Priapus. But I do not feel sexual right now. I am longing for the experience of soul."

The tree wants to get into this. "I am a palm tree and not a phallus. It is incredible how people cannot tell the difference."

The man asks the tree, "How does it make you feel to be called a phallus?"

"I know what I am, so I don't feel threatened."

The priapic interpreter now sees the woman's extension from the man's body as a phallic symbol around which his arms are wrapped.

The woman refuses to respond.

The man wants to speak again. "Sexualizing my desire obscures the deeper feeling. It is a bigger risk to dive into the feminine and acknowledge its presence in me.

"I am only beginning to see my lifelong pattern of overextension, overreaching, overdoing, overwhelming, trying too hard. The effort has always been extreme, pushing too hard, being too much, talking too much, wanting too much. The desire has propelled me through life, but it can be difficult for other people."

The woman is instructive. She moves in a way that is comfortable for her, and she is above him. She gently helps him observe his unconscious tension and effort. "Relax. Don't try so hard to control me and this situation. Let it all go and you will have what you need and shed the things that take too much room. And you will perform better!"

The male and female figures in this picture inhabit the same psyche. They are among its many aspects. It is tempting to take this scenario literally and conclude that control and exertion are masculine qualities or problems. Hercules and other mythic males throughout history have had their share of these pathologies. But psychic traits and emotions do not have genders. They inhabit people of both sexes and are not exclusively masculine or feminine.

Figure 7 is the first version of the man grasping for the woman. It is an oil painting made before figure 6, which is an oil pastel. The pictures illustrate how an image changes through repetition. The difference in

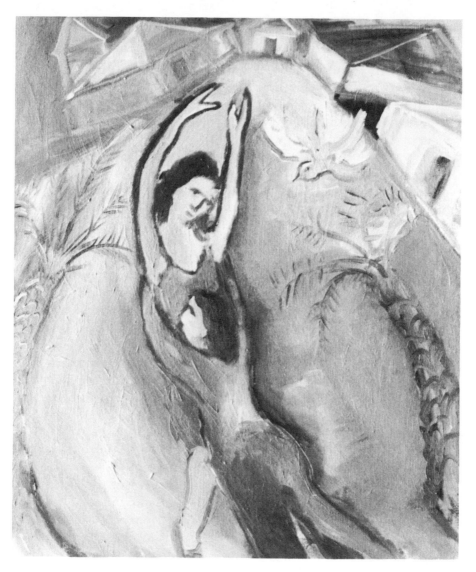

Fig. 7

169

the medium will alter the character of the image. This picture has a more dreamy and mysterious atmosphere. The space is misty and the boundaries are less distinct than in the previous picture, owing largely to the medium, the oil paint.

Let's consider similarities between figures 6 and 7. The man and the woman interact in both pictures; the human figures are in approximately the same place in each composition; palm trees appear in both images; in each picture the people are flanked by vertical forms—two palm trees in this picture and a palm tree and the red street light in the previous image; and each picture has at least one building with a simple doorway.

The woman's face in this picture is different. She does not seem to be floating away. Maybe he has a better grasp on her. But she is not concerned with escaping. Her arms are interacting with the surrounding space. There is less tension and more fluidity than in the previous picture, where the direction of the man's body is continued by the woman's arms, from the bottom right to top left. That straight, diagonal extension contrasts to the curve here. The woman leans into the center of the picture. Her upraised arms connect the figures with the buildings at the top. There is a sense of envelopment together with an upward movement. The man and the woman form one figure that sweeps up, and all of the movement goes into the tiny building at the top of the painting.

The tardis clearly appeared prior to my seeing it in my student's painting. The evidence is here and in other images in my studio. We were both making the same image. It came to both of us. Seeing the small building in her pictures affirmed its presence in mine. I became more aware of it. "Theft," originality, and the presence of autonomous forms seem to be secondary features of my obsession with this building. The primary concern is fascination with its visual qualities.

That little structure in this painting receives tremendous movement. It is barely discernible from the background. It was painted in quickly with a few strokes of the brush to fill the space. And now it has taken on great significance in the painting. Everything moves up and converges on the doorway in the distance—the figures, the palm trees, the buildings, and the colors.

There are two trees here, on either side, and they almost merge with the atmosphere. They are less distinct than the tree in the previous picture.

The presence of the bird sets the tone of the picture. It resembles the bird in figure 4. It is a gentle, fluttering bird that focuses on the two people, and it can be imagined as a guardian. The leaves of the palm trees are feathery and soothing, and they move like the wings of the bird. The atmosphere of the picture influences the interaction between the man and the woman. They are melting into each other. They express yet another aspect of the interplay between the masculine and the feminine.

In my pictures there are many recurring themes: the interaction between the masculine and the feminine; the emergence of the feminine; the palm tree; the Middle East; the presence of animals; the flying figure as an intermediary between the dreamworld and the painting; views from windows, which are recurring dream images.

Architecture complements nature and suggests the human presence. The passageways in this picture evoke the mystery of what is on the other side, what is inside. But "beyond the horizon" fantasies can take us away from this particular image.

I make buildings, rooms, and furniture in my pictures because I desire to work with straight lines and oblique angles, distinct contrasts to curves, spirals, and circular shapes. Architecture enables me to increase the formal interactions within the pictorial space. In this image it would be boring to have the figures ascending into sky.

Some art therapists equate straight lines with the masculine and curves with the feminine. I prefer not to assign genders to lines. These interpretations obscure their qualities and varieties. We have to be wary of our anthropomorphism.

Cities, buildings, and rooms evoke psychic interiority. They are psychological environments. There is an interplay between inside and outside. And architecture evokes history, delighting the soul with its spaces, vistas, adornments, and craftsmanship.

In this picture the architecture is simple and straightforward. Basic structures and designs do not interfere with the direct visceral expression of the paint. Simple structures interact well with the materials, and they allow me to work with expressionist textures, colors, and shapes within a figurative context. They provoke imagination and associations while at the same time offering just enough compositional variation to create a structural basis for the painting.

The buildings in this picture are a good example of the effort to simplify. If they were drawn with more detail, they would not blend with the atmosphere. Yet they also suggest a village, a community, human habitations.

That last statement aroused something in the buildings. "What makes you so sure that we are 'human habitations'?" they demand.

That statement emerged spontaneously to counter the association to buildings in daily life. The buildings are getting ready to talk again. Acknowledging their autonomous lives within the medium of the painting liberates *their* voices.

"Yes, you are right. You have to work at distinguishing us from yourself and your experience. We exist on the surface of this painting. There is nothing inside us. We have no meaning or purpose other than what you see in front of you. We are shapes, colors, thick paint on top of paint, lines, and movement. We are so many different things. The buildings are just the last form that the paint took within the movement of this picture. We are not fixed to the earth. The flights of imagination are closer to our nature. The 'mask' of the building is something we wear to stimulate your expression."

These flying buildings now look like a vortex, and everything is drawn toward the small one in the middle. The world is truly in flight when buildings move through the air as naturally as the white bird. Getting too involved with the literal idea of the "building" or "house" can limit the fluidity of the image. It is another form of labeling, a subtle one. Knowledge about houses, birds, human relationships, and any other element of the picture can stop the motion of the image. The picture exists within the reality of imagination and the medium of expression. All relations established with life outside its world are analogies. When we see that even the forms at the top of this picture cannot be reduced with absolute finality to the idea of "houses," the pitfalls of interpretive labeling become more evident.

Imagine the hierophants who will tell us that the doorways are vaginal openings that the man desires. There are so many of them here! Or they will say that the man's grasping of the woman around the midsection of her body is an expression of the artist's desire to return to his mother's womb.

The first of these interpretations stays somewhat within the context of the picture—the grasping man desires the feminine opening. The second interpretation leaves the image and makes a statement about the longings of the artist for the mother who is not present. These are interesting analogies and perhaps worth considering as imaginal helpers. But if we cannot say with certainty that the forms at the top of the painting are houses, then it would seem that any person who takes the latter interpretations as facts instead of analogy has difficulty accepting the realities of artistic imagination.

Interpreters are apt to make assumptions about an artist's psyche on the basis of one picture. Typically, less attention is given to a series of works. By showing a number of different pictures of the interaction between the masculine and the feminine, we see how forms of expression are always changing. As we continue to make art on a particular theme, varied aspects appear. All of these characters or emotions are present in the theme itself, and they emerge as a result of the artist's sustained attention. Artists have access to all of them. An individual picture within a series reveals a particular configuration of emotions. The image is an incident within the shifting play, or field, of expression, which is in constant transition. The passages may be abrupt or drawn out, and the quality of the movement is something for hierophants to consider in addition to categorizing pictures.

In figure 8 (page 174), I wanted to deal with flight, and I consciously reflected on how flying figures introduce movement and vitality to a picture. My paintings over the past few years are full of flying figures. I have not been consciously influenced by Chagall or other painters who represent psychic flight. I do fly overseas frequently to do my work with art therapy, and thus the shamanic metaphor of travel has an actual basis in my life.

Again the man is reaching toward the woman. That is indisputable. She may be the more elusive of the two. The animal is a strong and grounding presence in this image. Its legs go off the surface. The picture was made quickly so that the movement and thickness of the paint would be as strong as the figures. I wanted a vital sensuousness in which the figures interact with an environment of paint. The Middle Eastern wall is in the background. There are three stylized palm trees between the man and the woman. The trees were painted in the spirit of quickness and without concern for representational rendering. I was more interested in composition and motion. There are also three palm trees sitting oddly on top of the wall in the upper left section of the picture for the sake of design and movement.

Hierarchical thinking is discouraged by simplified presentation of the humans, the dog, the trees, and the wall, together with the thickness of the paint, the texture, and the presence of the reddish color in all

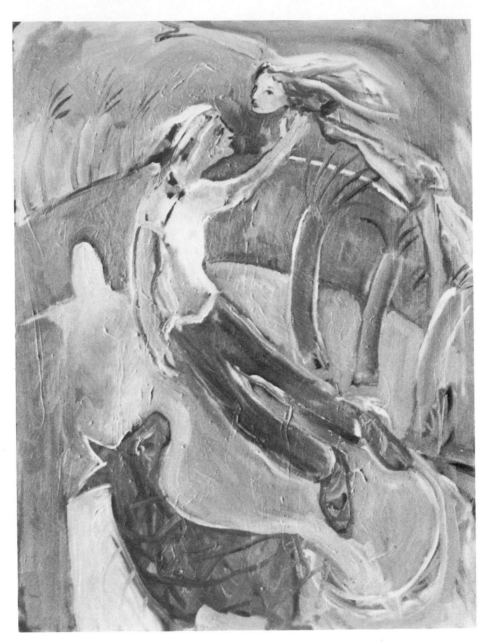

Fig. 8

sections. Every part makes its contribution. All of the elements are present, vital, and involved. There is no need to speculate on anything outside the context of this frame.

The vertical shape that runs from the bottom left corner of the picture to the midpoint of the left side appeared without intention. The picture was painted as a field of emotion where the interactions among forms, colors, and texture are as important as the telling of a story. The sensuousness of the paint is as important as the subject matter. The crisscross strokes across the dog show more interest in the paint and the design than in the dog's anatomy. Pictures take on emotions and personalities during the process of painting. Figures and environments acquire attributes through action rather than planning. They emerge through the successive strokes made on the canvas.

The dog is the solitary and reflective figure. The animal usually has this role in my pictures, especially the dog. It accompanies other figures and watches over them in keeping with the archetypal nature of the dog. Here it seems intrigued with the movements of the human realm.

The man is welcoming the woman, or what I have called the feminine. They are in their respective places. He is not overly eager, nor is she concerned about getting away. Her glance looks beyond him. They are comfortable, each floating in a personal space yet with the other. They are in a process of flight, and they imbibe the sensuous atmosphere, as in dreams and reveries.

Does the man have anything to say?

He reflects on how good it is to have a companion and how comfortable it is when they let each other be while also flying together. He looks at her and reaches to touch her cheek. He has an inclination to say something about how it feels to be with her; how fortunate he is; how he never tires of her tenderness and gentleness; how she renews youthful romance with its soft touches, sweet smells, timid movements, and pink moods. After arresting the sentimental clichés, he feels the urge to speak.

He smiles and says, "Did you feed the dog?"

She laughs.

What is she pondering?

She thinks, "I like him. I like him when he is this way. His body is relaxed and his eyes are comforting. He's not talking. He can get too serious about being romantic. He tries so hard to describe the feeling he is having that he stops feeling. When he jokes around, there is more flow."

The painting hangs in the most visible wall in our house, so it is a part of my daily life. It evokes feeling every time I look at it. The physical qualities of the paint correspond to the emotion I feel in the figures. When I made this one during the summer, I dreamed at night about paint. I applied thick oil paint when making this picture, and in my dreams I enjoyed the movement of the oils sliding across the canvas, the mixing of the colors, and the emergence of shapes from the free movements. There was no subject matter in these dream paintings, just paint. Psyche responded to the process of making paintings during the day with sensuous, nonintellectual dreams about the medium. This is one of the healing elements of art, the sensuous and direct engagement of paint.

Perhaps the colors, textures, and movements of this image remind me of the values and sensuous wonder that drew me to art as a life work. I have to continually renew my vocation and fall back into the grace of art. It is fascinating how easy it is to move away from this formative vision, and I do not want to lose my first affection for paint and color. This image joins an appreciation of soft colors with the need to be earthy and spontaneous. The thick textures are gritty, and this increases the appeal of the shades of rose color that pervade the picture. They are fleshy colors, and since I worked with thick paint and linseed oil, the moist gloss accentuates connections to interiors.

After I completed this picture, my art as a whole made a transition to spiral compositions in which figures and forms were shaped from thick, oily paints and motion. It was a period of liberation and delight with the medium. At that time I dreamt that *I am on the back of a motorcycle going through a field and down a wet path, through puddles* [it was raining while I was dreaming]. *I do not know who is driving the motorcycle, but I am relaxed. The motorcycle accelerates and flies into the air, does a flowing flip, and lands gracefully.*

I was stunned by how the motorcycle flight continued and transformed the euphoria I felt about the circular swirl in my painting. The dream and painting were paired in expressing the ecstasy of wet and streaking movements. This dream vivifies my idea of the shamanic machine. I also remember something James Hillman said to me about the James Dean flights of the *puer* archetype. Male sexuality is present in the surging bike, but I am more interested in the way the dream ego sits behind the "unknown" driver and lets himself be taken into flight. Giving up control and trusting the driver of psyche's motorcycle intrigues me. It fits and amplifies the emotion of the painting. Flight and movement for their own sake.

Figure 9 (page 178) is a recent painting on the male-and-female theme. The man plays his flute and the woman reclines. A bird is with them in the tropical environment.

The simple rendition of the houses is appealing. By abandoning the literal architecture and details of houses, they become aspects of the painted surface. The picture was made quickly, in about an hour and a half. Since there is emphasis on movement, texture, masses of color, and simple representation, the image has more vitality than a painting that strives for photographic realism.

The thickness and sensuousness of the paint and the picture's expressionistic qualities correspond to the previous image. Although the man, woman, architecture, animal, and palm trees are present in both pictures, the sense of subject matter in each is distinctly different. It is the bird who flies here, and the human figures are not only resting on the earth but are situated at the bottom of the canvas. The man is interacting with the bird, but he plays his music for all aspects of the picture, including himself. The woman peacefully gazes in another direction.

I painted the picture during the coldest time of our New England winter when my wife told me that she wanted a vacation in a tropical place. Although the picture was influenced by what happened between my wife and me, the figures that appear in the paintings are daimonic personages. I imagine all of the women in these pictures as devis, different manifestations and aspects of the psychic feminine. The same applies to the men, the animals, and nature.

Just yesterday we heard of the people who were killed when the Baghdad shelter was bombed. It is provocative to be looking at a pleasurable image during a difficult time. All of these moods and aspects are perpetually present in psyche, and consciousness shifts from one to the other.

In my early thirties I read *Moment of Freedom* by the Norwegian novelist Jens Bjørneboe. It reflects upon the history of human cruelty and evil, and I was struck by the way I had for many years overlooked that characteristic of the human psyche. As a child I was deeply compassionate toward victims of violence and vividly imagined what

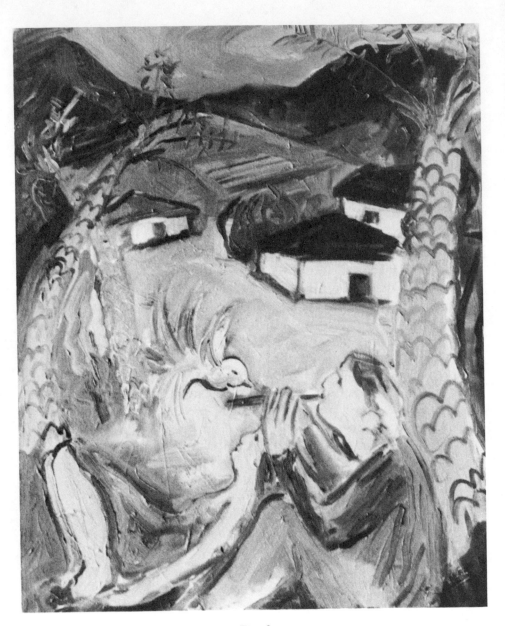

Fig. 9

they experienced. Bjørneboe says that power "means only one thing: the opportunity to cause others pain." History can be imagined as a constant cycle of cruelty. I have reestablished my childhood empathy for victims of violence, on whatever side they happen to be. I will often make a violent and aggressive image when these emotions grasp me or when they enter my sanctuary.

A moralizing voice inside me looks at this picture and says, "Why don't you paint pictures that reflect the suffering of the world? Your sensuous images are hedonistic. They are fantasies that deny the condition of the world."

And I reply, "Fantasy is a vital part of art and life. It is as real as the tortured and suffering souls you want me to face. I may be there sooner than I realize. Perhaps I am like an ancient Egyptian who feels that painted scenes will be repeated in the afterlife. But even if my life is sure to imitate my art, I do not want to live in an isolated paradise. Life is an ongoing moral engagement of the actual world, and I am refreshed by artistic reverie. I move in and out of it. The imaginal realm helps me to forget myself, to avoid taking myself too seriously, and to see myself as a character in imagination. I share your compassion for the suffering soul, but authoritarian commands produce zealots and puritans who oppress what does not fit their schemes."

I continue speaking to the voice: "Why do we have such a difficult time enjoying ourselves? Even a moral crusade becomes a grind that transforms itself into the energy it opposes. Reverie helps to ward off possession by unacknowledged aspects of ourselves that generate cruelty and evil."

"Do you mean that you have a cruel demon inside yourself?"

"Absolutely. I try not to project it onto others. The nasty characters are parts of psyche, and we are in psyche. This image of pleasure is part of psyche too. It may be more difficult for me to relax than grind it out for the commonweal."

There is another voice saying, "You are right on target now. When was the last time you sat down under a tree with your wife? Why don't you drop your work, your social work, and take her on a vacation?"

Zap! My ordinary pathology has been penetrated and uncovered. Crusades for the improvement of the world, as important as they are, can deny the need for a pilgrimage into the shadows of daily life.

I would like to go back to the painting. These deviations into morality have left it stranded and unattended. My talk may not have anything to do with the image, or it might have everything to do with it. Images stir the psyches of viewers in any number of ways.

My eye is drawn to the area of light between the buildings and the opening that goes toward the hills. My doorways are always open, and they lead into other realms. This picture speaks to me about the teeming richness of nature—the trees and vegetation in the foreground, the fields behind the houses, the movement in the sky—and the human presence.

The painting embodies my interest in psychic multiplicity. So many things are going on simultaneously, and no one is more important than another.

This image illustrates what I call the bioenergetics of painting. If we remove all references to subject matter and meanings and look at the painting only in terms of its physical qualities, we will enter the realm of its energetic patterns—thick textures moving in every direction, the bent palm trees, two of which crisscross on the left, the fast and thick strokes of paint in the bird's wings, the vegetation between the two trees on the left, the squiggles on the trees, the slashes of line that form their branches, the bold and straight lines of the houses, the swirling sky, the spontaneous fields, and the mountains shaped by quickly painted masses of dark color.

The interaction of varied elements within the image energizes me. I see now that the strokes of paint can be viewed as aggressive and bold, and this quality shapes my experience of the image even more than the romantic subject matter. So the picture is closer than I realized to the shadow aspects we discussed.

It is undoubtedly alive with varied qualities, and that pleases me. I am intrigued to see it evoking aggression, boldness, and the unrecognized underworld as well as imaginative reverie. It contributes to keeping the daimones alive.

Since we have focused so much on "romantic" themes, I would like to reflect on an embrace between a man and woman (figure 10). Actually the painting looks less romantic than the two previous images. It has an intensity that reminds me of Edvard Munch.

I wanted to make the figures merge. They have a youthful sincerity, a purity of emotion. There is an equality of stature. The woman might be smaller, but the effort of her reach and her illuminated legs complement the man's dark and firmly placed lower body.

She is on her toes, and her head reaches up to him with an extension of the neck. He is not as forceful, or perhaps he is pausing and looking. The containment of the couple within the relatively tight enclosure of the canvas surface and the snug passageway around them makes the emotion unavoidable and compressed. Downward movement is encouraged by the vertical shape of the canvas, the way their joined hands shape the arms into an arrow pointing down, the dark base, the suggestion of an archway above them, which closes off ascent. The necklines of their clothing similarly point down. The gap or hole

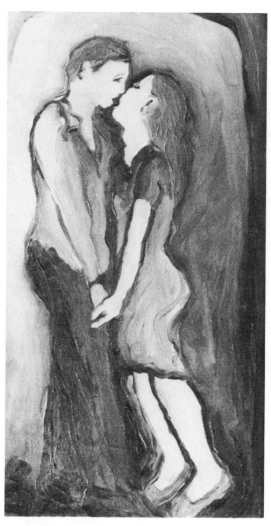

Fig. 10

where their mouths meet suggests yet another underworld opening. The mouths are not touching and seem to form a doorway between the masculine and feminine. There is a similar dark area or hiatus above the hands in the genital region. These qualities and the reddish environment in which they stand evoke primal emotions, extreme closeness, hunger, heat. There is a slight cooling and tempering offered by her blue dress and shoes and his relaxed posture. They press closely against one another at every point along the length of the body. But their hands are not clutching or grasping. She gently envelops his hand in hers.

Over the past three years my paintings have gotten considerably darker as I consciously engage the feminine. The darkness of color and environment came unintentionally together with dark openings. The emotional qualities of a painting may have more to do with the way paint is applied, colors, and environmental mood than with subject matter. The "shadow" may be expressing itself unconsciously in the way I apply paint and choose colors. This discussion helps me to see the feminine as part of my shadow. She is making an effort to become fully incorporated in the faces I show to the world.

Look at her here. She is going after him. He cannot avoid her. She is part of him and he is part of her. He looks completely open to her influence and passions. They are "psychic" twins, a pair. Their hair, skin color, and bodily features are similar. These figures are daimones, spiritual companions and intimates. The mixing of masculine and feminine instincts in the individual psyche might be a purpose of the frequent incestuous relations between deities in Greek mythology. The gods and goddesses are not to be taken literally as perpetrators of incest. They are personifications of primal emotions, and thus their behavior is rarely tidy and predictable. Rules that govern human morality do not always apply to figures of the imagination.

I do not identify with the man more than the woman here or in any of my pictures. I am recovering from the one-sided identification with the masculine that is stressed in the socialization of boys. Men's terror of identifying with the other gender can be an expression of our repressed and suppressed affections for men. The feminine gets mixed up in this. Identification with women is considered unmanly, and that is madness. The secure man can empathize with women and emulate them.

The two people in this picture do not have anything to say. They do not think. It is an underworld embrace, instinctual. Each person is enveloped in holding and desiring another human being. There is a loss of self that is blissful—one person's blood flows with another's. The pulses rhythmically connect in a primal life energy.

The last three pictures have something to say together: "We have been carefully constructed. Commitment and time have gone into creating us, and we want to speak as paintings through the sensuousness of the material and the suggestiveness of our movements and gestures. We want to reach you in this way. We want to arouse your senses. We want to enter you in ways other than your mind. We want to engage you without talk."

As I talked about dark openings and the feminine shadow in the last picture, I kept seeing in my mind the image that appears in figure 11 (page 184). Where the red, pink, and rose were subtle in figures 8 and 10, they are not here. There is nothing subtle about this one other than the gentleness of the woman's gesture and the animals. When I made the painting, those cavelike openings behind the woman were a major interest. They were intended to be doorways into primitive, earthen houses made with a curving line. There is a suggestion of a habitation, but the structures simultaneously function as pure form and color. The same applies to the tree on the right. The formal pattern of the buildings and their openings, and the contrast between the indigo and the Naples yellow, winds around the left side of the picture to the bottom. The blue animal is an extension from the indigo, looking at times like a pool of water.

The entire image swirls in a spiral pattern that recurs in my imagery. Over twenty years ago I made large paintings of lines, shapes, and colors, and I see that the motion and essential design here were the basis of pictures painted with a very different style and subject matter. Paintings that I made in 1969–1970 also had vivid primary colors. So there is a consistent kinetic orientation and boldness.

The vortex is a recurring pattern in my art and dreams, something that sweeps me into its world. This picture captures that movement. I get dizzy when I meditate on it. Even the large and apparently stationary cow on the right is part of the swirl. The fleshy red color above the cow is repeated below it, and there is only a slight contrast between the cow's colors and those that surround her. The absence of sharp differentiation takes the cow into the movement of the whole

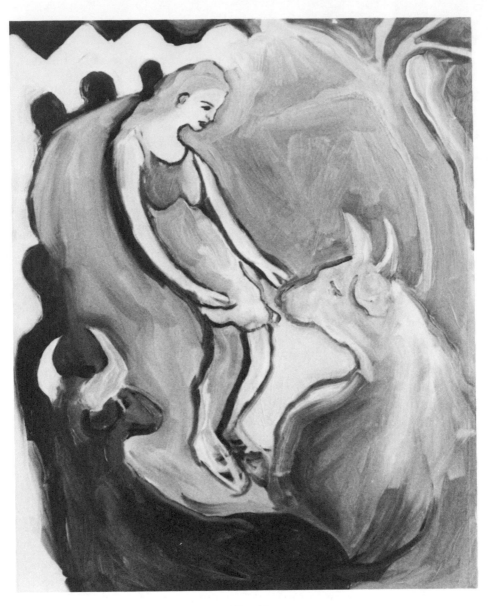

Fig. 11

composition. The same thing applies to the woman. Her dress combines the Naples yellow and the cadmium red that surround her, and her body is drawn with thick, indigo lines that relate her to the left side of the picture. Her body curves in sympathy with the context. The curvatures of the animals and the tree also further the circular movement of the image.

The spiral is often associated with life cycles, phases, returns, and renewals, and it is literally doing this in my art. It is remarkable to see how forms repeat themselves over time. Art therapy meditations make the connections. The spiral and vortex movements undoubtedly appear in the first movements that we make with paints and pencils as children. The movement patterns and the colors are the daimones who do not have fixed and distinguishable bodies. They are forces of involution that pull the painter into psyche. The woman in this picture is enveloped by nature and the animals. She spins in a theriomorphic and chthonic matrix. Creation is the deity here.

She is ready to speak: "I have got you now. I am not a figure inside you. You are beginning to see the way you have always been inside me. You did not go into established psychologies or religions or art movements. You are forever turning away from orthodoxies and doctrines in search of the inner movement, the pure kinesis of creation that leads to nothing but itself, to me. You are always after me, in devout pursuit of holy creation. You are just another brushstroke made by the eternities. This 'shadow' you talk about is the force of creation that you can never fully articulate, so you abandon yourself to it, your life and your ideas, you open and give up control so I can move through you and in you. These pictures do not look like images coming out of 'wildmen' gatherings in the woods. You miss all the movements, the women's and the men's, because you cannot look at one without the other, their interplay. You are more interested in letting it all go, all of the agendas, so there will be plenty of room for unexpected arrivals. You are becoming like the cow I touch. There is a sheen to your coat; it is smooth, not that tacky surface which holds on to everything falling its way. You dissolve, relax, and connect with the ground, your instincts, your sense of smell, your nose for creation. Meditate on the cows. They are your medicine."

The cow on the right wants to speak: "You are still loaded with energy, but you are more relaxed. Remember the dream you had a few months ago after listening to the lecture by the hyperactive young man who was full of himself? You felt bad for him because you sensed that the stories he told about his own importance were just covers for his insecurity. You understand that shadow self of worthlessness and the way it generates overactivity. You have been there.

"The figure in your dream who said, 'You've calmed down,' is a daimon of energy conservation. You see him now as the blue animal, the cool one here in this picture. You are opening to the grace of the animal life, sensing, listening, and paying attention to others. Maybe it is part of aging and the different seasons of psychic life.

"The wild and passionate movement is still here. Don't worry. It is in the dancing tree above me and in the colors and the sensuous shapes of this picture, the shapes between the figures, like the one between me and the woman's legs. You can shift this carnal aspect into the foreground whenever you want. Or it will come to you when it is ready. Right now you're interested in other aspects of life, in looking after others."

When I reflect back on poetry that I wrote years ago, the theme of spinning inward is constant. "I went to the navel of the world, Jerusalem, to find that there is no center, only motion, spinning rhythms . . . the spin that takes me in."

At that time, art for me was "a spinning transformer." Motion and intimacy were paired within the vortex.

The closeness of the figures in all of these paintings, and their sensuous movements, express a sense of divine life that embraces the physical and brings "the gods back to where they grew inside people" and between people and things. My shamanic interests emerged from the revisioning of a divine life that exists in all things, "a prairie of passion ready for the torch." It is spinning inside this image of the woman and the animals. The painting, in keeping with these earlier lines of poetry, captures an unconscious religious history "spontaneously from the body it sings."

Figure 12 is another painting of the woman and the animal. It was made before figure 11, and the figures emerged from large and sweeping lines on the canvas. The woman, tree, animal, and building are parts of a circular configuration. The picture was painted quickly. It expresses pulsating vitality rather than ethereal spirit. I am attracted to its boldness, dark lines, thick textures, movement, the intimacy between human and animal realms. The tree on the right looks like a shamanic creature, and whenever I meditate on that figure, the painting comes alive.

I remember another line from one of my poems from ten years ago:

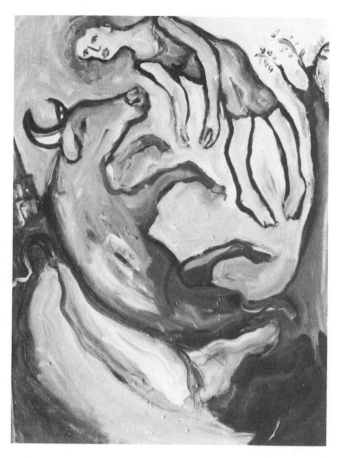

Fig. 12

"Spin, spin, holy spin. Sit still and you'll never get in." Stillness has its place, of course, but my daimon prefers Mick Jagger, rolling and spinning. This woman's big red lips look like his. Soul is kinetic, rhythmic, palpable, the vibrating earth. I want to follow its most vital paths, which are usually labyrinthian, spirals and spins, seldom linear. The painting is an icon containing these forces.

Samuel Beckett ultimately discovered that the darkness that he fought was his subject matter. The same applies to the religious doctrines that repel me. The struggle against religion is a relationship to it.

I see how inflexibility motivates expression. My friend Truman Nelson said, "Find the breaking point, the point of revolution, change, and transformation." But this cannot be a search for something outside our experience. We have to find it in ourselves. The woman and her blue animal could be a transformation of my intimate relationship with the Madonna. The real religion is what we do every day, the life we are living and do not see. I find myself living this unconscious or unstated religion of spinning movement, emerging images, intimacies, and primordial longings.

A Freudian says, "You are really longing for your mother and you suffer from your separation from her body. That loss is at the root of it all. Your spiral movements expresses your wish to return to the womb, where you were nourished unconsciously like this animal."

I reply, "Perhaps, but don't be so simplistic and trite. It is vaster than my mother and me and what we used to be. And your explaining leads nowhere. The care and love that a mother gave is part of the spiral, the movement. I do not long to return to a fixed place in the past. I am interested in a moving vitality that is stimulated by memories. You literal-minded Freudians cannot see that I have never left the feminine and her mystical body. I don't have to return because I am always in it. The spiral enclosure is not the literal body of my mother. It is a cosmic womb."

After all this reflection on spinning, I looked at a series of pictures that I made in an art therapy studio not long ago that focused on the theme of "shamanic washing machines." In those pictures I wanted to make something private and very ordinary. Computers, automobiles, and other mechanical artifacts have become part of our psychic lives, yet we are generally unaware of their contributions.

Figure 13 was made in response to these reflections on machines. The woman in figure 12 interacts with the blue animal, and the woman in this picture comes out of a bluish washing machine. The womens' bodies in both pictures are in similar positions and are located in approximately the same zone of the circular compositions. This image was made some months after figure 12, and there were no conscious connections. I did wish to admit the technological dimension into my psychic environment. I wanted to express the most common aspect of my daily life through the washing machine. The container of Wisk and the clothes on the line came in response to the laundry motif.

The devi comes right out of the machine, out of the ordinary. Or perhaps she goes into the machine, which opens to other worlds, travels, transformations, and cleansings. The mundane artifact is imag-

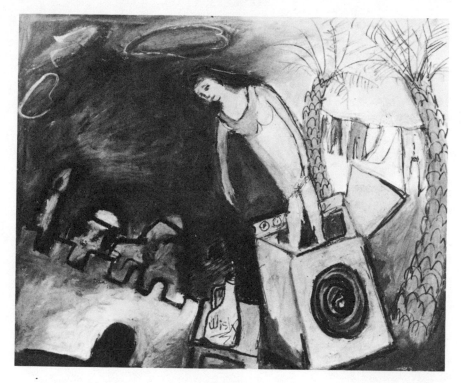

Fig. 13

ined as an instrument of passage rites. As Jung said, "The savior is either the insignificant thing itself or else arises out of it" (1958, p. 120).

My artistic figures live in laundry rooms instead of on Mount Olympus. Yet I do locate this laundry scene in an environment with my omnipresent palm trees, Middle Eastern city, and red clouds. My painting studio at home is in a room where we do our laundry. I sit right next to the washer and dryer when I paint.

This picture and the one that follows are illustrative. I imagine them as part of a shamanic storybook. The washing machine woman says, "I have come to help you renew your vocation, your devotion to the commonplace, to the sacred routine, the overlooked spirits. The mysterious city is right under your nose, the eons are inside you, inside the spinning of my machine. Yes, those building tops are phallic. The Wisk container is too, the cleansing 'agent.' Don't be afraid of them. Take your masculine attributes along. They are part of the spin, the 'wisk,' and moving city. Nothing stands still.

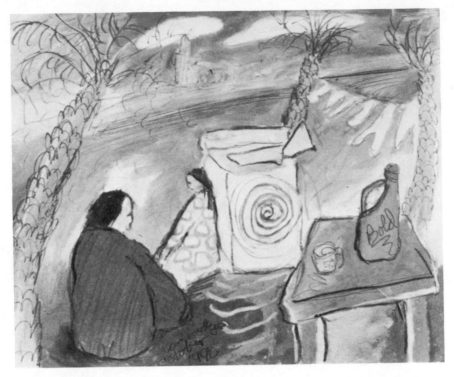

Fig. 14

"You are smiling. You think it is funny, to replace Botticelli's sea shell with a washing machine. I am the Venus who lives in your machines. Don't take them for granted. Don't disparage the machines as you use them. Thank them for the work they do. The deities live in ordinary places."

The Native Americans fit into figure 14 because it is an imaginal world, more open and relaxed than the previous picture. There is a sense of hiatus. The sky is green, and the wind is blowing the clothes on the line between the two trees on the right. The men express the sacred realm, classical shamanism, and ties to the past. Although the washing machine with its spiral window is in the center of the picture, it is the jug of Bold on the red table in the lower right that is the most significant object for me. When I made the picture I felt my interest move away from the washing machine and toward the table with the detergent on it. The ordinariness of the Bold container is attractive.

Yet it is potent, phallic, "bold." It repeats the curved vertical movements of the palm trees and relates to the tower in the distance. The circular cup with its small spiral echos the spiral in the washer.

As I reflect on the picture I am carried into the central spiral in the washing machine. The Native Americans look like attendants who are meditating. The red table is a place for ritual objects.

This process reveals my idiosyncrasies, my odd nature. The confession urges the soul to speak. The picture says, "Every day you have sacred connections to the objects in your environment, but they are unconscious. You walk down the stairs in a daze, looking at the dust on the windowsill; you open the door for the dog and feel the cold and stand there watching his black muscular body run through the woods; you go back inside and move toward the sink, turn the faucet, fill the kettle, and make a fire; you sit there looking at the woods; and you wait for the urge to either paint or write. You have arranged your life so you can sit and experience these things rather than rush out for early morning appointments. You are a crazy guy because you take these things seriously. It feels mad because no one else is doing it. You are a man of odd combinations—washing machines and shamans.

"Many years ago you started to see that it is all a matter of days following days, routines and changes, with the treasures inaccessible to those who try too hard to get into the sanctum. You wrote a long poem called 'Each Day.' Do you recognize these lines?"

> & day upon day just a matter of
> either you are, or are not
>
> all gradations between
> nothing but abstractions
>
> in the circle going nowhere,
> just breathing days. . . .
>
> where each day is a volume of *Ulysses*,
> celebrating instants . . .
> that dissolve
> and fade with the sounds in the air . . .
> where soul's viola is silent
> and revives
> in a frenzy of IFs leaving footprints on the water.

I thought I was through with this picture, but the expansion of expression occurs when we shift from literal to imaginal discourse. I relearn this principle with every image. The voice in the dialogue retrieves aspects of life that are so distant that they seem to have been written and experienced by another person. I change over the years and each day. I can even feel myself change within the shifting moments of this dialogue as different themes appear. This shamanic washing machine spins an unexpected tale. As I let myself enter its world, the poetic labyrinth flourishes. The washing machine comes to spin me into imagination's voices that the psychotic takes literally and the rationalist disparages.

And now the superego judge says, "You should be more active in the world and get out of your private environment. Enough reflection! More achievement!"

I become anxious about the value of my life.

An ecstatic voice revives itself and declares: "Life is a *Kunstgarten*, and as Blake says, 'All that lives is holy'—even the washing machines and the Bold detergent. I am caught by the need to have the time to reflect on the life that happens each day. Deep down is forever right now. No other time will do. It cannot be postponed. 'If not now, when?' I marry moments and die with them. The deity is in the things we do and the objects we touch without thinking. The divine is that creation that we make without knowing, every day, day after day. The unconscious purpose is in ordinary life, ordinary objects, everything we do. Goethe said, 'What is the hardest thing of all? That which seems the easiest for your eyes to see, that which lies before your eyes.' The simpler, the deeper. The holy land is everywhere. Let's not pass by the full moon of our bodies."

The thoughts are spinning like the spiral in the washing machine. It is getting abstract as the feelings and inspirations are conveyed through words. I paint pictures to meditate on objects, colors, and physical things. Making detergents and washing machines into sacred artifacts shows that everything counts, nothing is eliminated from the circle.

Now a "green" voice enters: "You are a polluter if you use Bold. It is full of toxic chemicals that you put into the earth. And you appropriate the Native Americans with your rituals."

I reply, "Don't you see that it would be corny to make a picture of Native Americans with just sage and other 'pure' substances? They are in this mechanical world too. You suggest that people who have lived close to the earth have something to teach us about what we put into her. When you become the voice of authoritative commandments, the big voice speaking from the green sky of this picture about what I should and should not do, the imaginal birds fly away. You stop the process. I have to protect this picture from you. The Bold container feels rejected, guilty about its provocations, its bright red color. All of expression's creatures have their significance in art. You and your opinions and concerns for the world, your greening, are welcome as players within the imagination. You have already touched me with your compassion for the earth. I see the dark green around the table's legs for the first time. And the bright blue to the right of the machine supports your purpose."

Dialogue continuously opens new views and possibilities, like a dream of going to the top floor of a familiar house and discovering rooms with sweeping views of a blue sea, delighting in new rooms and vistas. The same applies to dreams that affirm the darkness of the underworld by presenting rooms under rooms in the cellar of psyche.

Last night after writing about shamanic washing machines I dreamt that *a short and stubby old man runs a race with young people and surprisingly leads until he is unable to run anymore. Then the dream shifts to him looking at an image of a Pan figure with a head like a boar and feathered legs. As he continues to look at the image, he begins to resemble it.* At first I felt that the shamanic daimones came to tell me to stop being playful and blasphemous about them with my laundry imagery. But I see that our fears and guilts stop us from going further. As I reflect on the complete dream, the inability to run encourages the inward meditation of the Native Americans in this picture. When the aged man can no longer "run," he meets the extraordinary shamanic creature, and as he studies the figure, he starts to resemble it. Life is shaped and influenced by images of imagination.

There may be no message in this dream and no message in this picture. The figures are complete unto themselves, and their purpose may be nothing other than engagement for its own sake. "Communication" is only one of many aspects of expression. Yet it tends to monopolize the psychological industry. We "read" our dreams in the morning rather than meditate on their mysterious music.

The desiccation of living experience through analysis is an old problem that is itself part of psyche's archetypal pathology. "Tables

Turned" by William Wordsworth illustrates the malady and the artistic
medicine.

> Sweet is the lore which Nature brings;
> Our meddling intellect
> Mis-shapes the beauteous forms of things:
> We murder to dissect.
>
> . . . .
>
> Come forth, and bring with you a heart
> That watches and receives.

There is a correspondence between this poem and the dream that I
just described. The old man with arrested movement is transformed
when he "watches and receives" the extraordinary creature. Unable to
move, he opens to imaginal Nature and is changed into a new life.

Aesthetically I like figure 15 more than the washing machine series.

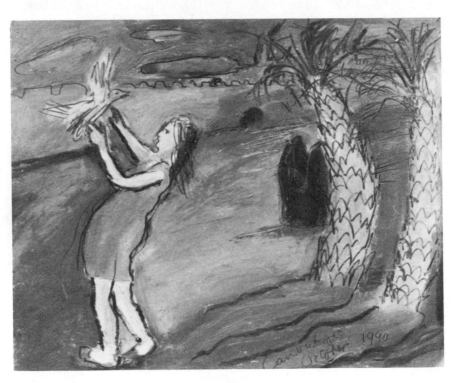

Fig. 15

The color, the mystery, and the way the figure interacts with the bird keep my attention.

The city is decisively walled, and it runs across the entire surface of the picture. There is a sense of divisions, but I do not feel exclusion. There is a large opening in the wall, and I experience the city as a place where these figures can go at will. The wall and the black opening create mystery. The group of black figures seems related to the black opening. They are stationary as contrasted to the movements of the bird and the figure. The dark earthy colors and especially the deep green sky with smoky red clouds evoke a somber mood, which makes me increasingly curious about the figure with the bird.

The omnipresent palm trees are protectors and witnesses. They watch and receive, as Wordsworth suggested. The trees show no bias. Their sensitivities extend in all directions. They do not experience the linear perspective of the human. Their senses are circular and absorbing. Their branches reach into the air and their roots into the ground.

If I look at this picture within the context of right now, rather than try to recall feelings while making it, the bird comes to the woman, who also looks like a man, to encourage flight. Or perhaps the human figure releases the bird and lets it follow its instincts for movement and survival.

The three black figures are obscure and turned into themselves. There may be more people whom we cannot see because of the tree. These figures are an expression of mystery and subtle suggestiveness. Simple black shapes without detail can express distinct feelings. The contained grouping is intriguing. They communicate with each other while the viewer and the figure with the bird are outside their sphere. Perhaps they are members of a tradition that does not look outside itself. Their lives are enclosed within the frame of their beliefs. They turn their backs to the action in the foreground, whereas the figure on the left faces the bird and opens to it. The position of the body with its upraised arms and curved posture is responsive.

The figure reaching toward the bird says, "I have an impulse to touch you and hold you, but I know that I cannot. You are a wild creature. I am attracted to you, but I do not belong with you. I do not belong with those people in black either. They accept me and I contribute to the life of the community, but I do not feel that I am one of them. I cannot accept the restrictions of their beliefs. Every form of life intrigues me. I am attracted to every new bird who flies into my life."

The bird replies, "I sense that you are fascinated with flight. You are ready to take off. You go between worlds, the city and nature, the new and the established. I am the moving soul that you try to hold and cannot touch. But you do not envy my ability to fly, and you see it as part of my nature. You are preparing for psychic flight, which is part of your nature. I am an imaginal bird. I can be your intimate, your bird spirit. I bring no messages, only myself and spirit's flight."

The figure speaks again to the bird: "I was feeling isolated and depressed before you came. I have been alone here, and nothing significant seems to happen. These feelings result from living outside the enclosed community. It is hard to avoid intimidation when I compare myself to other people who have a definite role in their group. They do not have to choose what they do every day. Their lives are completely organized by their environments. I cannot accept this for myself, but I see its value. My feelings of worthlessness are an expression of egocentrism. Your presence is the only thing that matters right now. You fly out of depression."

The tension and struggle of the previous picture are gone from figure 16. The person is clearly feminine and relaxed. The colors are soft with cool, blue mountains, purple below the woman, and a purple door in the small building which returns to its place outside the city. Her dress is a soft and nourishing green. The black dog looks like a shadow. The city has a wide and welcoming opening in the center of the picture. The small building looks like a guard's shelter on the outskirts of the city. The woman's feet connect her to the building, and yet she is not isolated from the city. The whole environment is an imaginal scene where everything belongs.

Now I see the small building as a portable shelter, something that provides comfort and continuity for expression as it visits exotic environments. It houses my psychic familiars. They travel in it. The small house is not a stationary or permanent abode. It functions as a charm, evoking imagination wherever it appears. Everything is relaxed and accepting. The lack of tension in the woman's body sets the tone. But she seems focused on something below her. The dog is also alert and points outside the picture. I imagine the dog welcoming guests, the next phase of the creative process.

Flight liberates the figure, and it offers the medicine of air, imagination, and movement. This flying figure relates to every aspect of the composition and is not identified with one place on the ground.

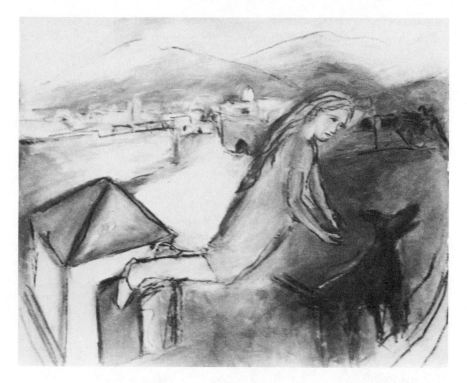

Fig. 16

The woman reflects, "Everything in this environment is with me. It is crazy how quickly the imagination shifts from isolation and depression to ecstasy. The weather is always changing. I am able to fly when I forget myself and my preoccupations and when I feel grateful to nature and imagination for whatever appears."

A voice from somewhere says, "Now you are on one of your manic flights. The shifts you talk about are called manic-depression. You are 'a manic.' There is no mystery, just chemistry. Be careful about celebrating this illness. You are contributing to madness. If your fluctuations get severe and disturbing, we have a drug that will keep you balanced and on the ground. Our pills will fix your problem."

The woman responds, "No, thank you. This condition is not something to be fixed or even balanced. Moods are the winds that propel my flight. Fluctuations of emotion involve me in all of psyche's aspects. I cannot experience one without the others. I admire people who fully experience an emotion and go on to another. I respect chemistry and its dream of transformation. It is your psychology of control and chemical management that concerns me. You assume that your drugs will bring me to a better condition, whereas I want to perfect the art of living with what appears."

The woman in figure 17 reflects, "I live by the sea where the tides

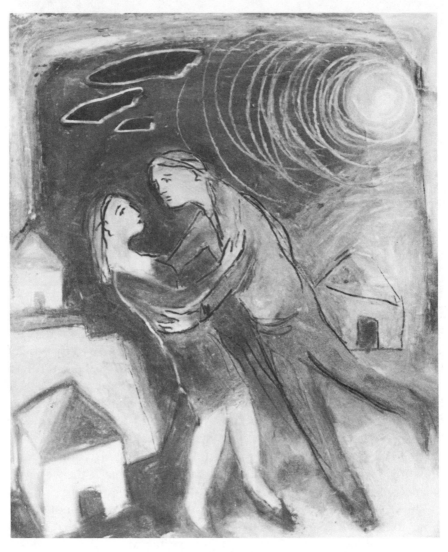

Fig. 17

teach me about high and low water, ebbs and flows. I trust that fulfillment and perfection will come in their time, together with disappointments. This man came during my flight. He is not permanent, and I will soon pass from this moment with him to yet another phase of travel. But I am going to enjoy him while he is here. I can let him go because I trust that he will appear again. My disappointments and my struggles contribute to this glow."

Considerable effort went into making this picture. I struggled with it and painted it over and over again, knowing that it could be ruined by excessive effort. The thickness of the oil pastels ultimately supported the qualities of fantasy and atmosphere. At one point it was too complex, and the only way to solve the problem of composition was through radical simplification.

After many failed attempts, the small buildings that envelop the couple came as a solution, affirming the trust that the woman described.

The houses look like stations of an artistic process. I imagine an endless series of them.

The emotional weather continues to change. I cannot cling to the peaceful moment that I saw in the previous image. The small buildings in figure 18 (page 200) support the fantasy I had about stations along the route of the artistic journey.

My pictures are stations of psyche, and the process of dialoguing enables me to stop and reflect along the way. Stations suggest travel and the way one art experience leads to the next.

I am not saying that these small buildings are now "stations." Metaphors quickly and unconsciously become literal. While I was meditating on the three buildings in the previous picture, the idea of stations emerged, and I extended the metaphor to the individual pictures that I make. The image was so appealing that I expanded its reference from the buildings to everything I do. Today I imagine my life within the metaphor of stations, and tomorrow it will be something different.

There is no contradiction in the pictures. They are decisively themselves, evoking different voices and feelings.

Are these shifts a sign of pathological fragmentation? I do not think so. They are manifestations of different voices and feelings, changes and movement from one condition to another. As I said previously, contradiction is a vital aspect of psychic reality. Contradictory conditions exist simultaneously within us. I experience grace as the ability to flow from one to the other. I strive to perfect graceful movement rather than acquire a substance called grace. Experiences are temporal but movement is eternal.

Here comes the chastising voice again, "I am tired of your blasphemies. You take too many liberties with religion. You know what the stations of the cross are. You know the suffering they embody. Why do you appropriate them into this business about shamanic and artistic travel? And grace does not belong here. Its nature is defined by religious doctrine."

I reply, "As always, this conflict with you clearly defines differences."

"Please, do not go into your 'process' talk. Speak to the issue."

"I have to reimagine and refresh sacred notions to feel their life. The divinity speaks to me poetically, through metaphor and images. One of my Jesuit professors used to speak about the 'heresy of literalism.'

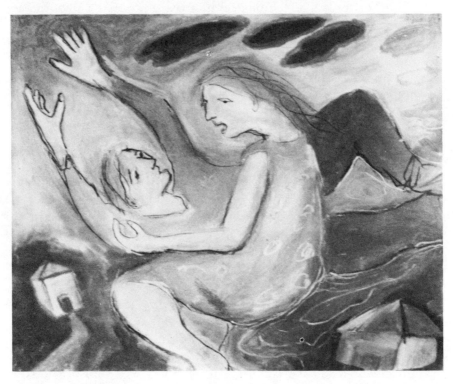

Fig. 18

Reason is to be cultivated for what it can do, but it can go only so far. I feel grace in creation, and experience its absence in doctrine."

We have left the picture before us. Talk about religion will do it every time. This is why meditation on art is such good medicine, even for religion. The physical presence of the image treats the tendency to fly off into opinions and indefinite things. When I look at this picture, it cures me of intellectualizing.

Unlike the one before it, this picture came together quickly. Struggle led to catharsis. One condition feeds the other. Liberation in painting frequently follows an accumulation of tension, and the force of the release is influenced by the degree of the conflict. Spontaneous pictures are often triggered by frustration and anger. Prolonged dissatisfaction with a picture can be a preparation for a new eruption. Or, as in the preceding picture, the result can be a more systematic simplification.

Let's return to figure 18. The two figures are in the sky where the man expresses the soothing effects of release.

He says, "Letting go is euphoric."

I do not find this picture disturbing. It is comforting. Strong feelings are being expressed. But we can easily shift to a man in a condition of need, expressing resignation and helplessness, while the woman supports him.

The roles again can change as quickly as the emotions, and he may find himself comforting her. This interplay between feelings is at the heart of the labyrinthian journey. The small buildings again become expressions of travel, the shifts that I have described from one place to another. I am fond of them and their simple contributions to this picture.

The man and the woman talk at once. He says, "Would you let me be? Let me fall. Let go of your need to care for others. Relax. I have to do this alone. I have to spend time with myself and feel the isolation. Please don't touch me, not now."

Simultaneously, the woman says, "I am afraid to be alone with myself, so I am always taking care of people. Helping others affirms my existence, my worth. I cling to your needs."

Psychic life is a movement from feeling to feeling with all of their diversities coming into play. Art's medicine affirms the shifts, the aesthetics of travel, imaginative engagement, and letting go.

Let's completely restate these interpretations of the picture and see what happens.

The man and woman are now incapable of talking. They make primal sounds and flow with the elements. They are only small parts of nature but in this instant their concentration on each other fills their immediate space. I experience grace in his resignation and her compassion.

The two small houses below ponder in unison, "We are here for them. We are safe and separate places where they can retreat to listen to their individual natures in silence."

Someone asks, "How does your talk about angels and daimones relate to pictures and dialogue?"

I reply, "The words accompany drawings and paintings like angels."

"You sound tentative."

"I have an urge to say 'as angels,' but I cannot make an absolute or positive statement about what an angel is. The pictures are saying, 'Angels are not required to have wings.' I agree. Angelic images are not restricted to winged and fair-skinned humans who wear pastel robes. My vision of the words or pictures functioning as angels is a personal statement. The image of the angel will be something else for you. It is a protean force."

"Do you disregard the classifications and hierarchies of medieval angelology—the seraphim, cherubim, thrones, dominions, virtues, powers, principalities, archangels, and angels?"

"No. They are expressions of the medieval imagination that still live. But if angels are going to be alive for me, I have to envision my personal relationship to them, and theirs to me. The medieval tradition may influence me, but my imagination prefers a more archaic daimon, and it engages the poetic, mercurial, and personal nature of the angel as a presence that takes varied forms and performs many functions. My vision of paintings and words as angels expresses a desire to connect imagination and the world. Everything I have done in art therapy is part of this *imago* longing for cooperation between art and life, between words and pictures, between imagination and the suffering soul."

"You want to revive the function of angel as messenger."

"Yes, art works carry messages, but they are not just messengers. Rather than saying that the pictures 'are' angels, I am more comfortable suggesting that they are analogous to the figures of imagination that we call angels, who emanate into distinct 'persons' through creative expression. These personages do not always have human charac-

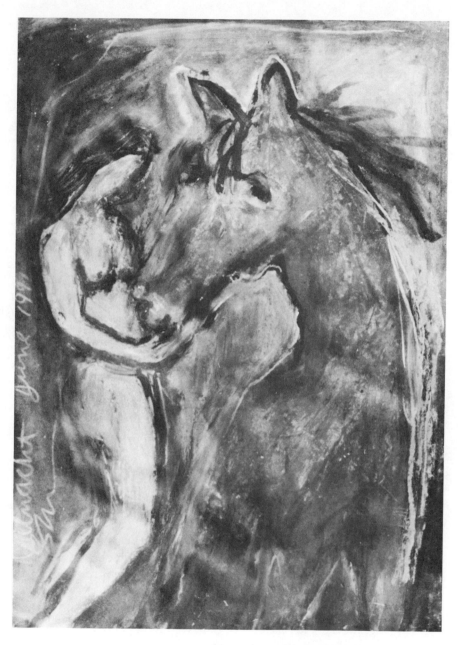

Fig. 19

teristics. They include textures, shapes, lines, colors, and other qualities of pictures, which function in ways that are analogous to tutelary spirits, familiars, and guides. Angels offer another angle on art."

The questioner continues to confront me. "You avoid definition again by making analogies."

I respond, "Imaginal reality is metaphoric and analogous to existence in the physical world. Analogy is a link between imagination and the world. It connects the inner and the outer without compromising their respective natures. When I say that a painting 'is' an angel, I take away the latter's invisibility. Analogy enables the picture to function in an angelic manner without limiting its ability to do other things. Analogous connections maintain fluidity."

Let's talk about angels in relation to figure 19 (page 203).

I have been skirting eros in our talk about war, religion, and washing machines. This picture evokes sexual aspects of eros. It was made in Switzerland after I took a walk on the mountain during a midday break in my studio work. It was the first week of June, and the farmers were cutting hay in their fields. In the Appenzell region, men drive the tractor that cuts and bales the hay while women walk behind with large wooden rakes gathering what remains. Typically the women wear long cotton dresses and cover themselves from the sun.

It was a hot day and the sky was clear. I came to a field on a steep incline and saw a couple working. He was on the tractor and she walked behind, dragging a rake in the traditional fashion. But she also broke the farm tradition by wearing a loose tank top and what must have been a tiny bikini bottom, gathered between her buttocks. Her legs were muscular and very white. It looked like a pastoral setting from a D. H. Lawrence painting.

I imagined the young woman irritated by the conservative Appenzell culture where until recently only men could vote. "If you want me to pull this rake behind you, I will show my behind to the world, whose eyes will follow me," she might be saying.

It is more likely that the Swiss woman was just uninhibited in showing her body. Her irritation is my fantasy, and my eyes were probably the only ones that were arrested by her image. Whatever her motives, the scene I saw in the field lodged itself in my imagination. My ruminations were not devoid of sexual feeling, but my principal response was idyllic and full of feeling for the primal relationship between humans and nature and our animal instincts.

The derisive voice says, "You do not have to justify an erotic feeling."

I reply, "The image appeared like an angel. It had many aspects—sexual, pastoral, angelic. Ancient religions celebrate all of them, whereas Western indoctrination sees the devil in sexual imagination. Our repressions have actually stimulated devilish fantasy."

The voice continues, "But enough comparative religion and fantasy. I want to hear more about this picture."

"I returned to the studio and felt the scene would lose imaginal vitality if I tried to re-create it. I made quick-gesture drawings of figures in black ink. This image emerged from one of the gestures. At first it was a genderless figure standing next to a horse. When I started to work on it with oil pastels, it became more sensuous. The horse is deep red with blue highlights. The woman is faceless, as contrasted to the well-defined head and snout of the horse. The horse's neck, his or hers, is phallic. The woman cradles the snout in her arms, while the midsection of her body and her pelvic area lean toward the animal. I thought of the woman in the field while I was working on the figure's thighs and buttocks, and I realize now that I never saw her face. Anonymity and darkness affirm instinct. But the scene in the field was in the full light of day."

"You draw the pastoral scene into the underworld," the voice says.

"I have dimmed the lights and obscured the face. This picture begins with my feelings about the scene in the field and creates another life, probably in response to the black ink I was using. I do not want to limit the freedom of the picture with suggestions that it does not adequately represent the situation that helped to stimulate its creation. The final picture may actually have little to do with the scene in the field other than the fact that I returned to the studio with strong feelings about what I saw: I wanted to make a picture immediately; I decided not to represent my memory of the scene; I scribbled figures with black ink, and this composition emerged."

The dissatisfied voice says, "I am confused about why you relate the making of the picture to the fantasy of the farm scene. What do they have to do with one another?"

"Eros was stirred by the walk, and his energy was concentrated in the making of the picture."

"Sublimation?"

"That is a characteristic of what I am describing, but the moral emphasis of sublimation, the channeling of the feeling into a 'socially acceptable' expression, turns the psychology of art into a process of secondary substitutions. Eros was aroused during the walk and emerged in this picture. The 'primary' process was continuous from episode to episode. I am trying to describe how a feeling finds its way into an artistic expression and how it is continuously transformed as it moves. Morality is one of many collaborators in that the feeling has a sensitivity to others. As a personified figure, the feeling is less likely to be motivated by a singular moral imperative."

"You said you were going to relate this to angels and daimones."

"As I talk to you, every one of the figures in my memory and the figures in this picture are increasingly animated. They function as angels or daimones. They are so alive within my imagination right now that I have left the rational context from which I discussed them earlier."

"They 'are' angels rather than being analogous to them."

"Both," I say. "It depends upon your perspective, whether it is imaginal or rational."

I am tiring of description and am eager to hear what the figures have to say. No doubt I did more explaining than usual because of the sexual aspects of the image. The embarrassed voice in me anxiously says, "Let me explain. Please let me explain!"

And I reply, "No. Enough. The image speaks for itself. Please step out of its way. It does not want to be obscured by explanations. The eros in the picture and the sexual fantasies that visit do not belong exclusively to the artist."

The horse speaks immediately. "I am red and vital but I do not feel sexual. So relax. Do not excuse your instincts. That offends me. Celebrate what you saw and felt on your walk!

"I like the way the woman touches me. I am comfortable with her. She is a soulmate. We are a pair within this image, complementing each other. We are in the eros of nature, the sensing of color, light and darkness, texture, touch, closeness, and the shadow between us."

The woman says to me, "I do not have a face but I am full of feeling. The face of this horse looks like you. We are your familiar figures, the feminine and animal instincts."

I see a kinship between myself and the horse's face and body. The horse embodies the carnal existence that the woman in the field arouses in me. She expresses an ideal, the human body as a sentient figure in the field of nature, the eros of nature and place.

The harsh voice returns, "You are using all of this talk and sentiment to cover your identification with the man driving the machine. He is on his seat, and the woman walks behind as an extension of his world. The story that you do not tell reveals the appeal of the scene. You have not said anything about the man and your masculinity. You go on and on about women and animals, avoiding and denying your real agenda. Your picture shows this. The horse with your face is in the foreground, and it is attended by a faceless woman."

I say to the harsh voice, "Why am I so stimulated by your way of talking? I like the way you confront me, turn tables, shift perspectives, and temper my romantic and compassionate inclinations. You must be my shadow voice, the one I do not use outside intimate relationships, where I have used you blindly, ventilating and exercising your sharp edge. You help me to see that playfulness and letting the nasty characters speak through imagination brings them out of the shadows. The theater of dialogue affirms the expression of our repressed voices without getting entangled in them. The livelier the better. Have your say. Let the contraries exist."

"You sound like William Blake in your euphoria, and you are slipping away again with your affirmations and compliments. You avoid the content of my observations when you speak about the 'process' of conversation."

"I heard what you said and I accept it as a response. We are in an ongoing conflict about meanings. There is no single reason, no exclusive determination about what the picture means, no absolutely 'real agenda' other than the dialogue itself.

"Defensive statements are unattractive to me, but since you press me, I will try to clarify how I feel about the man sitting in the tractor. He is not in my picture and I do not identify with him. He is a footnote, a supporting actor to the image of the field. The history of my relationships to women is not directly relevant to this picture or my fantasy about the woman in the field. I have never had a woman walk behind me with a rake, and to the best of my self-knowledge, I have never desired that type of relationship with a woman. In my psyche woman is primary and not subservient.

"There I go talking about my history when I just said it was irrelevant. Positive statements always assert their contraries. I took the bait and began to recite boring defenses. Moralizing lacks imagination. Your confrontation is a no-win setup if I take it literally. If you say the 'real' story is the one I do not tell, everything is undermined because the supposed reality does not exist. What happened here is that you told another story about the man driving the tractor. Rather than going into the imagination of that story as an independent thing, I got caught in your successful attempt to attribute its origins to me. I could have played with the story, but instead I 'explained' how it has nothing to do with me and embroiled myself in it. I tried to present myself as a good guy, and my wife came in and told me she just had a dream in which she walks behind me carrying bags of groceries."

The provocateur replies, "Isn't the shadow the part of yourself that you most vehemently deny, the unattractive trait that you work so hard to correct with good works and noble intentions?"

"The way I leaped to the defense and lost my playfulness does say something to me about my shadow, the man on the tractor that I called a 'footnote,' the one I did not put into the light of this picture. Perhaps he is in the dark area between the figures. But if we separate this image from my psyche, if I can forget about myself and my moral critics, the man who was sitting on the tractor did not seem the least concerned. He was doing his work. That particular image does not have to be corrected. I was sidetracked from protecting its integrity by your innuendos about my finding that scenario attractive. You touched a sensitive spot, and I made myself, and my shadows, the issue rather than the image. It is all part of the action and the ongoing distinctions.

"You may be onto something about my masculinity. I have not even replied to that aspect of your question. The next image speaks to the theme of the large woman and the small man."

Figure 20 was made in Switzerland immediately after the picture of the woman and horse. It also emerged from a fast sketch in black ink with a wide brush. The woman is large, powerful, and grounded. She extends from earth, whereas the small, timid-looking man is in flight. The bird and the small building accompany them and help to complete the composition. The picture pleases me aesthetically. It has the bold and free qualities of working quickly, with the body leading and the mind tagging along, or flying like a bird accompanying the hand.

I see for the first time how this image expresses the spontaneous "flight" of the hand that made the picture. It is a stunning revelation because I had not seen how the picture is organized around the hand and arm. It was apparently so successful as an instinctual process of movement that it has taken me this long to see the contents that correspond to the way the picture was fashioned. The composition is an homage to spontaneity.

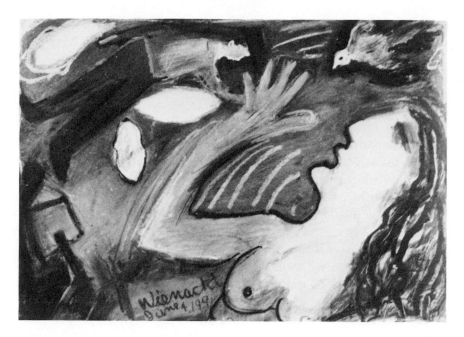

Fig. 20

The size of the woman is consistent with my descriptions of the feminine aspects of creation. The man is there but he lets himself fly. He gives up his need to be in control. In this picture I see him as whimsical and youthful, and the absence of facial features says something about his ability to be inconspicuous, a supporting player.

People in my studios during the past year have been making crosses, which have intrigued me. I scribbled one in quickly at the bottom left. It looked incomplete, so I put a quick feminine loop at the top of it.

The woman appears hermaphroditic. She has a hard and prominent face and a genderless arm. The small figure that I called a man looks less masculine as I speak. I see its feminine aspects—the gentle face, the petite chin and nose, the long hair.

I was all set to use this picture as evidence to support the suggestion that I have to affirm the masculine. I began to imagine a new series of paintings of men.

The human figure in the previous picture is beginning to look masculine, and the horse seems more feminine with its big eyes and long soft hair. The "unspoken" perspective turns out to be the hermaphrodite, not the repressed masculine, which keeps us in dichotomy.

All of my pictures can be imagined as expressing the hermaphroditic mixings of creation, Hermes and Aphrodite. If I obey the directive to work on my masculinity, I become a servant of the dualistic consciousness. I lose the feminine as a primary and formative partner. The two aspects are forever interacting and taking on different roles in relation to each other. Art's purpose is stifled by simplistic dichotomies about masculinity and femininity. The hermaphrodite of creation is closer to soul's condition.

The lines and colors want to speak. "Do not forget about us. We are becoming lost in the talk about hermaphrodites. We are the forces that give life to this picture. The figures on the surface are illusions, recognizable forms we took to please and intrigue your eyes. Motion, strokes, and layers of matter on paper are the primal nature of this picture."

The artist replies, "You work together with the imagination of the figures. I see you as partners. The figures emanate from your motions, and the emerging composition influences later gestures."

There are many different strokes in the picture. The six quick lines between the large figure's arm and chin were the last marks I made. They are the signature of spontaneity. Each one is a being, a part of a group that sets the tone of the image. The same applies to the scribbled handwriting at the bottom. And they were all created in an instant, without planning.

The six lines say to me, "You are getting tangled in calculations that can't reveal whether your masculine is less active than your feminine or vice versa, and there is no perfect balance between the two. You meditate on them to experience their mysteries and not to perfect your balance sheet. Stop measuring and don't worry about your masculinity."

"I dealt with the masculine in the chapter on dreams. I am covered."

"There you go again making a defense by trying to balance everything. Stop computing! Your vitality is in this picture. It is neither masculine nor feminine. You are not afraid of being soft. It is the other way around. Our forceful directness is your dominant style, and neither trait has a gender. Don't be confused by bossy voices telling you to do something contrary to your nature. You exemplify the neurotic process of trying to anticipate how to act according to the changing standards of moral 'correctness.' Listen to your instincts and spontaneous intuitions. This picture affirms their presence."

Figure 21 (page 212) brings illumination and spaciousness to the interaction between the woman and the animal. Turmoil, conflict, and sexual energy are not in the picture.

Eros is present without sexuality. The colors, figures, and textures of paint are sensuous and pleasing to my eye. The paint is thick and was applied quickly. The woman's gesture is so simple and pure that it borders on cliché.

A voice emerges now from the picture. "Look at me and let go of your desire to say something deep and profound.

"Do you enjoy me?"

"Yes."

"That is enough."

The woman laughs and smiles. She continues, "I am a presence in your life. Just accept me. You men find it so difficult to see your feminine angels. It doesn't have to be so complex. I am here together with the animal, the paint, and the gestures of this picture."

Figure 22 (page 213) continues the meditation on the presence of eros in the nonsexual spheres of life. The two women act separately, but simultaneously, and this corresponds to my sense of what happens most of the time in domestic situations with other people. The figures appear to be involved in the basics of daily life, whereas the environment through the large window, or door, is unusual. I imagine balmy air, a fertile Mediterranean region that corresponds to my image of Lawrence Durrell's *Alexandria Quartet*. Although the room in which the figures stand is intimate, there is a large opening to an expanse. The pervasive pink color connects all parts of the image, so there is a permeability between inside and outside.

The trees contrast to the demure women. Although their ecstatic blossoming can be seen as male exuberance, they make more sense within the painting as a passageway, a natural archway between the opening in the foreground and the rounded opening in the wall. The regal palms soften what would otherwise be a sharply angular and austere space. They are intermediaries between the room and the city. The location of the trees creates a converging perspective from the foreground to the opening in the wall and the imagination then moves through the spaces beyond.

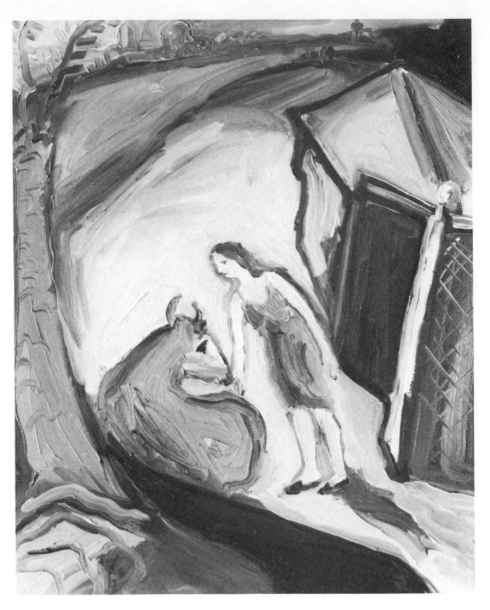

Fig. 21

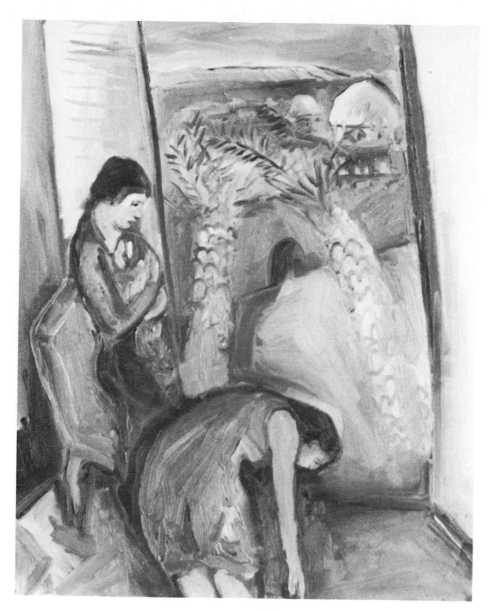

Fig. 22

If I had looked at the trees exclusively as phallic figures, I would have missed these spatial and aesthetic features, which feel closer to the soul of the picture.

Sexualizing the image is always an interpretive option. I can easily shift to the perspective of the trees as an expression of bursting male desire, waiting outside the door, while the women are interested in other things. However, I am annoyed by interpreters who assert that the picture is always expressing unconscious sexual conflict. Eros is present in every element of this picture, and it would be repressive to limit its place to sexuality. I feel eros in the air, the distant hills, the earthen walls, the shadow, the touch between woman and child, the paint and colors, the foreign setting. The sexual aspect is always present, latent and ready to emerge, but it is not in the foreground of my imagination of this picture. Other qualities of eros evoke my interests, especially the sensibility of space and the way in which Arab civilization has contributed to this aesthetic.

The picture expresses the place of eros in domestic life, a physical and aesthetic appreciation for everything we do.

There is a mystery as to the nature of the relationship between the women. Are they sisters? Friends? A nurse and a housekeeper? A couple? If we leave the imagination of roles, then the figures are simply present together, two women in close proximity. The need to attach clearly defined roles to them expresses an inability to stay with the mystery.

The figures perform instinctual and unconscious actions while expressing how two people can be together and at the same time separate. They do not appear to have needs to control one another.

I am asked, "Is there a particular quality of the picture that provokes these emotions?"

"It is the sense of domestic intimacy," I reply.

"Between two women?"

"Intimacy makes itself available to any combination of figures."

"But in this picture you painted two women."

"The female figures are manifesting themselves clearly and consistently within these paintings."

A Jungian analyst smiles and says, "Your anima exudes from the pores of the painting—in the women, the pervasive pink, the nurturing of the child, the openings, the city, the palms, the landscape—your domes look like breasts."

I smile at the analyst and reply, "Yes. The idea of anima, the man's unconscious femininity, is helpful. This picture and others in the series present her in many different ways. She cannot be reduced to one thing like sex differences, which keeps us in oppositionalism. Hermaphroditism is not the single answer either. Hillman talks about how she is beyond all categories and definitions, the primordial 'life behind consciousness,' which is the source of all expression."

The women in the pictures say, "Wait a minute. We are not *yours*. You do not possess us. We are not manifestations of 'your anima.' "

"Thank you for this distinction," I reply. "Yes, you do not belong to me, and the same applies to masculine or animal aspects that appear in paintings. Will you accept the possibility that you came through me and that we are intimately connected to one another?"

"Yes. We feel traces of your sensibility in us. We emerged from your inward reflection and from the context of your life. Your feelings reflect the movements of our feminine soul, which cannot be possessed by a single person. We interact with you, and the specific qualities of this picture emerge from the movement."

"Anima manifests herself through my imaginal expression. I feel her presence in these paintings. They are not feminine parts of myself, but a feminine force that moves within me. Anima is an autonomous psychic force that can never be a part of myself, but I can become more aware of her presence, the way in which she influences me and my pictures. She cannot exist without this freedom. As soon as I begin to see one image as her definition, she protests. She must be free to move and continue her work."

A Freudian analyst enters. "Don't you see how all of this mystical talk of anima is a defense against your confusion about your sexual identification? Look at yourself in the women in this picture, in the baby being held by his mother, in the picture's romantic longing and nostalgia for enclosure in the feminine body."

I reply, "I accept your fantasy as an aspect of these anima meditations, which welcome every sincere contribution. She is especially hospitable to confusion. Her realm is outside the limits of conceptual definitions. Your certainties are a defense against her limitlessness."

"But what about the concrete forms of this picture?" the Freudian asks.

"They are the specific persons through which she is manifesting herself at this moment. If we go to another picture, her form will change."

"It's all you, not her, or that's the problem: you do not know what you are."

"Didn't you hear what the women in this picture said? They do not belong to me."

"Now you are saying that the pictures speak. You promote psychosis. It's only your imagination."

The women in the picture say, "Arguments about the nature of reality overlook our presence, our reality. We are no longer present in this picture; our imaginal reality leaves when it is seen as an extension of the man who made it. We are a presence in your life. Just accept us. Yes, we are related to the artist who made us, but we are not human. We lose our psychic identity when we are seen as parts of the artist. This subordinates us to him."

James Hillman enters and says, "Humanizing slays the animals, the *daimones*, and the gods. It turns the sacred *numinosum* of an archetypal image into something safe, sane, and secular. Man becomes the measure and the gods aberrations."

The Freudian says, "You are all deranged from the religious opiate. Look at the human forms in this picture!"

The women reply, "Of course we are related to humans. We take on their forms. But we are reflections in the medium of art and imagination. We are artistic angels, companions for those who are open to our reality. The extent to which we are present depends upon the quality of your meditation."

The dog, the woman, and the doorway converge toward the imaginal city in the distance (figure 23). The picture brings a feeling of repose and meditation. Relaxation is furthered by the open space, the light, and the absence of conflict. Even the paint is applied in a smooth and nonturbulent fashion with a light gloss. Yet there is a mood of expectancy.

The picture evokes feelings of receptivity and openness. But again I do not want to label these traits as feminine. They are aroused by the demeanor of this particular image of a woman.

There is considerable room for unexpected visitors, but I do not experience the woman as waiting. She has no agenda outside the context of what we see in the picture. She sits and watches, contemplating the illumination between herself and the city's labyrinths concealed behind the walls.

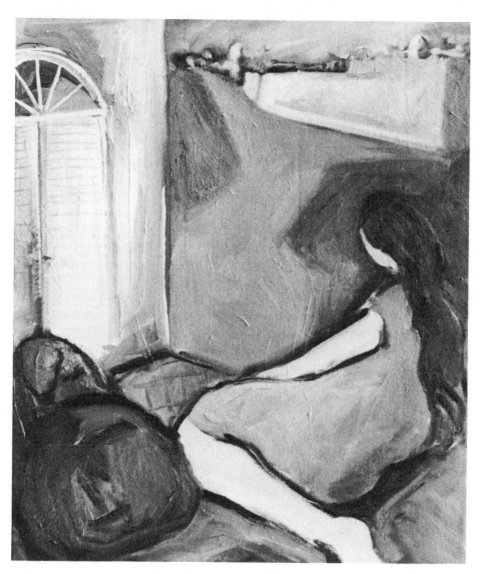

Fig. 23

The woman speaks: "How can you say that I have no agenda other than what you see in the picture? You may have no other considerations, but I am reflecting on the dream I just had. It is early morning and the city is asleep. Please do not assume that your thoughts correspond to mine. The city is a reflection of my dream with its varied passageways forgotten behind the walls of the waking mind."

Another voice says, "The woman's position resembles the reclining form of the cow in figure 21. Is your image of the feminine cowlike?"

I reply, "Of course not. The woman, the dog, the cow, and the men I have painted in similar reclining positions all express the gesture of repose, which does not have a gender."

I continue, "After all of this painting and dialogue, I had hoped that you would see that a similarity between the postures of a woman and a cow does not *mean* that the artist's image of woman is cowlike. You demonstrate how interpreters see a similarity between two figures and use it to make a declaration about the attitude of the artist who painted them. The cow is a cow, and the woman is a woman, and they happen to share a similar gesture in these pictures."

"But sometimes a cow is more than a cow and a woman is more than a woman."

"I know some women who will be offended by your suggestion, and the cows may not be comfortable in your presence. I see now that you are never content with something as it is presented. It always has to be 'more' than it appears to be. Latent meanings and hidden fears are your interests, your reality. I can accompany you in these reflections and enjoy them as long as you do not use them as replacements for the actual contents of the picture. It is the assumption that the true reality is the hidden one that offends me."

"You are the one who is fabricating these conflicts."

"If you and our culture denied covert meanings, I would surely take the other side. Psychological pluralism and the interplay among positions are my foundations."

"You need the argument."

"I apparently crave the friction, and I need a social purpose or cause. For more than twenty years I have been involved with the problem of people labeling pictures. It is never finished. My career has been constructed around the issue. Someone is always trying to say that a painting says this or that about the artist, and I jump in as protector of the image and explicator of the process of interpretation. I should give thanks to the pathology of attaching labels for everything that it has generated. The labels are tangible and provocative. They stimulate lively discourse."

The negative voice returns: "You are getting the picture. It is rarely the way you think it is. You are confessing a fascination with the psychological labels you oppose."

"I cannot deny that I am paired with this shadow aspect. We are partners of a sort. It does activate me and guide me, albeit negatively. I will confess that it has been my most consistent motivator. It has drawn out resources that I never knew existed."

Our psychologies reveal the pathologies of the collective mind. Imagine someone believing that a picture of a rainbow represents the artist's Oedipal conflicts. The desire for certainties creates the insane illusion that reason is in control of destiny. We veil life in explanatory fantasies.

I enthusiastically and graciously say "Thank you" to all of the interpretive confabulators, labelers, and their fleet of diagnostic tests, handbooks, and outrageous statements about the motivations of artists. They are my creators. Conflict invigorates and mobilizes dormant resources.

The reclining woman in this picture has been sitting quietly throughout my harangue.

She reflects to herself, "His defiance is the crusade he thinks he needs. I am here with the animal and the city of imagination to introduce him to a tranquillity unrealized. He thrives on having complaints. I can show him other ways to flourish."

I reply, " 'A tranquillity unrealized.' She arouses my curiosity. There is a confidence in her stillness. I will return to this picture and continue to meditate on its tranquillity."

I referred earlier to painting this woman over a pack of wolflike animals and leaving the one red hound on the right (fig. 24, page 220). The palm trees exude life and fertility. The bird arouses her and flies into consciousness like a thought.

Maybe she is giving birth, with the bird and hound acting as attendants. But the wolflike animals gave birth to her, and they serve as her underpainting. She is the "new tranquillity" that has been suggested to me. She is the metamorphosed state of wolflike energy that is still part

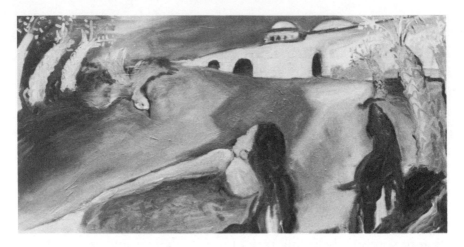

Fig. 24

of her being, something she can draw on if necessary. One alert hound remains as a helper and companion.

The picture says, "Lie back and relax. Changes and creations will appear in their time. This is a fertile place. The trees and animals are brimming with life."

I am not one to lie down in the face of challenge. Although she is reclining, she has considerable authority. She wisely and instinctively conserves resources.

She says, "You can be a vital player without leaping to attention. Watch. Listen. Wait. Act when you are needed."

There is the lesson of a lifetime in her last statement. Jumping into conflicts with good intentions and a sense of authority about what needs to be done usually fuels the chaos. The mess is passed on to the self-designated saviors. Contribute and step aside.

The man has returned. He is a humble supplicant who recognizes his daimon, the animal guide to instinct and imagination. Figure 25 returns to the man with whom we began in figure 1, the one who bends to the ground in the presence of animals, praying, contacting the earth.

The city is an interpretation of Bethlehem. I was not consciously making a religious comment. I liked the look of the city. But there it is, the birthplace of a religion. Yeats's poem "The Second Coming" comes to mind. I am intrigued by the poem's explicit connections to this picture.

The darkness drops again; but now I know
The twenty centuries of stony sleep
Were vexed to nightmare by a rocking cradle,
And what rough beast, its hour come round at last,
Slouches toward Bethlehem to be born?

I do not see the man "slouching" toward the city. He is already there in the company of phallic towers, bold lines and colors, and the

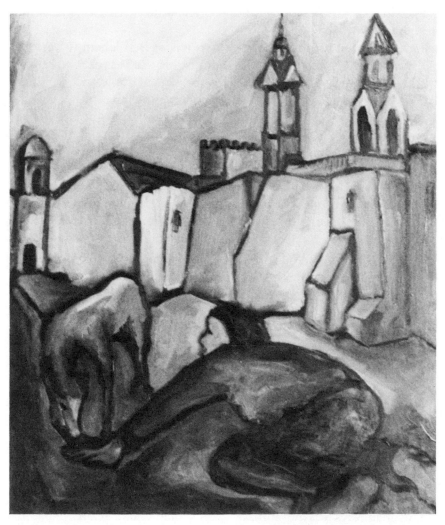

Fig. 25

sentient animal. The earth is a bright cadmium red. It says, "You have to get off your feet to feel my vitality. You engage me through your knees and the palms of your hands."

I want to shift away from the sanctified perspective. It feels superficial.

The man is looking for something. He says, "Where did she go? I am alone now. No, she has transformed herself into this red earth, the visceral world."

The animal sniffs the ground, which still carries traces of her presence.

Earlier I was caught in the "big" symbols of Bethlehem towers and walls, conflicts between religions, nations. I looked at the picture for a half-hour and felt stuck. The walls were impenetrable and the doors closed. By going into the imagination of a vanished presence, I was not engaging what is present. No doubt I had to let "her" go. The hiatus, or pause, was needed to make a transition to the vitalism of the picture.

The colors and bold gestures say, "You tell your therapy students that they have to let go of the person they just saw in order to open to the one before them. How can you miss our sanguine hues, riotous pigment, forceful and confident lines! Don't try to make us into something other than what we are. You are so involved in the woman's message about 'unrealized tranquillity' that you have lost contact with your other qualities. Haven't you been saying that people are multiple and never singular? Tranquillity alone is not the prescription. No one said this soul work would be easy and simple. Tranquillity can coexist with your boldness.

"Forget about the stories you have been telling and the preceding dialogues. 'Remember' this advice whenever you are blocked in your creation: 'Forget!' Don't try to connect things and fit everything together, especially at the end of the book. Please, no attempts to wrap it all up. That would be a denial of everything you have said about spontaneous arrivals. Work with the conflict you are having. Even if she has been transformed into color, you approach the red as though you are speaking to 'her,' and you miss 'its' nature. The dog is trying to tell you this. Sense the colors for what they are and don't use them as substitutes for something that is gone. Soul is always the immediate environment. You cannot hang on to the past."

The man says to the animal, "Let's play," and realizes that his statement is inappropriate.

Bethlehem is not a playful place today, and I do not feel frivolous looking at this picture. My feeling corresponds to the Yeats poem. My wife keeps saying that she likes the painting, and I find it disturbing. I just read through the earlier dialogue and I am touched by the line, "Where did she go? I am alone now." This emotion suggests that although I have to let the past go, the emptiness can be disorienting and the loss may sidetrack me for a while. The situation evokes unconscious emotions associated with loss. The particular instance is obscured because of the way it triggers the accumulative condition of the emotion. I can see how the process works in a situation where the feelings are relatively mild like this one.

The feeling of my statement about being alone did not sink in when I first made it. I was too involved with the transformation of the woman into the red earth. Now a distinctly different feeling comes and it suggests why I find the picture disturbing. There is a surplus of male energy in the city. Once again dialogue takes me to bedrock emotion that I did not previously see.

The red earth is now analogous to the ache. The animal comforts the man. The woman is gone. The country is gone. The people are gone. The walls look like a prison with their bold, black, vertical lines. The entire picture is loaded with color, packed with feeling.

If I enter the imagination of Yeats's poem, the man is in the phallic and stony city with his animal guide. They are there to revive the red earth, whose hour has come. His statement—"Where did she go? I am alone now"—takes on a new significance within the context of the poem. Being alone prepares him for the new birth. I imagine the rough beast as the man in this picture and not the animal.

"The Second Coming" is frequently interpreted as an apocalyptic prophecy. Even if we experience the poem as a portent of destruction, the decomposition generates birth, a second birth. The beast "slouches toward Bethlehem to be born."

I am becoming fond of the picture. These reflections, or amplifications, place it in a mythic and dramatic context. My previous uneasiness was related to its directness and raw emotion. Some people find my paintings too strong, too visceral, and I may have been looking at this picture through those judgments. Shall I accommodate my expression to what other people like? I have internalized this conflict, and it interferes with the way I relate to my pictures. Yet I know that soul prefers unusual, strange, and bold expressions. I strive, often unconsciously, to individuate my expression, and this instinct conflicts with public taste. Soul is esoteric and private, not public. Perhaps soul wants the images to stay peculiar and I am in a struggle with this wish because I want people to enjoy my pictures. One sees radical peculiarity in the art of mental patients, and this accounts for its appeal to me.

If we are painting for soul, our pictures will often appear "strange."

The animal asks, "Have you overlooked my aggression?"

The intense colors, and especially the red earth, suggest the presence of aggressive powers. I do not see manifest aggression in the animal, but it is no doubt there if needed. I am intrigued by the way in which the animal's mouth and the man's hand interact. In the picture the feeling is calm. I had a dream in which *I put my hand into the mouth of a red retriever* [a normally gentle breed] *and the dog digs its teeth into me. I become angry and try to pry out my hand, and the dog bites even harder.*

"The scene is calm now, but it can change in an instant, like my moods," the animal says. "The force in the color and lines can change directions quickly."

The emotions will never let go of their grip on us. Animals teach natural coexistence with instinct. The man in this picture is on all fours, resembling the animal. Rather than disparaging the animal as a lower life form, this man enters the animal's world to relearn its instinctual wisdom. It is in the instinctual realms where we humans make such a mess of the world.

The work with the previous picture shows how I can lock onto a theme that has passed. The block to creative feeling was trying to tell me, "Let it pass and go on to the next one. If you must, embrace the problem."

The solitary man is meditating on the work he has done inside the Yankee house (fig. 26). The oak tree is a link to eternities. With deference to this legacy, he sits in its shadow. He is the servant of a vision, and another phase of labor has been completed. The inverted table is empty because he does not want company at this moment. He wants to sit with the stillness of completion, the emptiness that comes after expression.

He says to himself, "I have nothing more to write. It is time to regenerate, work in the garden, paint the house and some pictures. I feel comfortable here, but I do not know where I belong. I do not know what to do, so I sit. I have never known where I belong, so I work with whatever presents itself and follow the lead of instincts and respond as well as I can. I occasionally initiate, but my expressions are usually responsive to the other, to the world, to the movements within myself."

The man continues, "It was difficult to talk with the last series of pictures. I am depressed—*post partum*. The project is telling me that it is over, and I have lost the daily purpose, the task, and the companionship, so I sit here and welcome the loss. It is the lost soul, the soul of the finished project that leaves me and, I hope, moves on to others. I am through with it and will go on to another task and a revival of soul. I am familiar with this emptiness. It is not new. It is the hiatus that separates, and leads to a new hunger, new stirrings.

"I do not want to think about new projects right now. I will sit with my feeling. Maybe this is how the 'unrealized tranquillity' begins. Depression acknowledges that loss. It is remarkable how still the emotion is. I feel inconsequential. The acorns will be dropping soon, falling everywhere, and new ideas will crack out of them."

I leave the man with his feeling. Instead of trying to help him cure his depression, I shift perspectives to the picture as a whole.

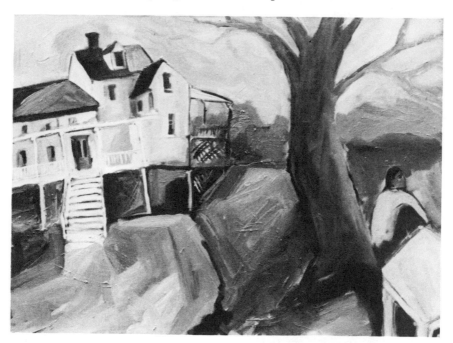

Fig. 26

The atmosphere of the painting is bucolic. The house and property are inviting and restful. They say, "This is a place of regeneration. We will take care of him. In a short time he will be active again. This depression slows him down and shuts off his creation for a while. He purges, lets go of inner involvements, mourns their loss. It is part of his preparation, his way of 'going on to the next one' and reengaging the world."

Bibliography

Alderman, Harold. 1977. *Nietzsche's Gift*. Athens: University of Ohio Press.

Apollinaire, Guillaume. 1956. *Oeuvres Poétiques*, ed. by Marcel Adéma and Michael Déraudin. Paris: Gallimard.

Arnheim, Rudolf. 1954. *Art and Visual Perception*. Berkeley and Los Angeles: University of California Press.

——. 1971. *Visual Thinking*. Berkeley and Los Angeles: University of California Press.

——. 1989. *Parables of Sun and Light: Observations on Psychology, the Arts and the Rest*. Berkeley and Los Angeles: University of California Press.

——. 1992. *To the Rescue of Art: Twenty-six Essays*. Berkeley and Los Angeles: University of California Press.

Balakian, Anna. 1947. *Literary Origins of Surrealism: A New Mysticism in French Poetry*. New York: New York University Press.

Barfield, Owen. 1967. *Speaker's Meaning*. Middletown, Conn.: Wesleyan University Press.

Breton, André. 1969. *Manifestoes of Surrealism*, trans. by Richard Seaver and Helen R. Lane. Ann Arbor: University of Michigan Press.

——. 1972. *Surrealism and Painting*, trans. by S. W. Taylor. New York: Harper and Row.

Burkert, Walter. 1985. *Greek Religion*, trans. by John Raffan. Cambridge: Harvard University Press.

Cavitch, David. 1985. *My Soul and I: The Inner Life of Walt Whitman*. Boston: Beacon Press.

Corbin, Henry. 1983. "Cyclical Time in Mazdaism and Ismailism" (1951) in *Man and Time: Papers from the Eranos Yearbooks*. Bollingen Series XXX 3, ed. by Joseph Campbell. Princeton: Princeton University Press.

——. 1988. *Avicenna and the Visionary Recital*, trans. by Willard R. Trask. Bollingen Series LXVI. Princeton: Princeton University Press. (Original French publication 1954.)

Dickinson, Emily. 1943. *The Poems of Emily Dickinson*, ed. by Martha Dickinson Bianchi and Alfred Leete Hampson. Boston: Little, Brown.

Eliade, Mircea. 1964. *Shamanism: Archaic Techniques of Ecstasy*. New York: Pantheon Books.

Ellmann, Richard. 1988. *A long the riverrun: Selected Essays*. New York: Alfred A. Knopf.

Ferm, Vergilius, ed. 1945. *An Encyclopedia of Religion*. New York: Philosophical Library.

Ferrini, Vincent. 1976. *Selected Poems*. Storrs: University of Connecticut Library.

————. 1991. *This Other Ocean, Books VI and VII of Know Fish*. Storrs: University of Connecticut Library.

Gadamer, Hans–Georg. 1977. *Philosophical Hermeneutics*, trans. and ed. by D. Linge. Berkeley and Los Angeles: University of California Press.

Hamilton, Edith, and Huntington Cairns, eds. 1961. *The Collected Dialogues of Plato*. Bollingen Series LXXI. Princeton: Princeton University Press.

Harrison, Jane. 1962. *Epilegomena to the Study of Greek Religion* and *Themis*. New York: University Books. (*Epilegomena*, first ed. 1921; *Themis*, first ed. 1912.)

Hastings, James, ed. 1928. *Encyclopedia of Religion and Ethics*, vol. 3. New York: Charles Scribner's Sons.

Hawthorne, Nathaniel. 1904. *The House of Seven Gables* (1851). Boston: Houghton Mifflin.

Hellman, John. 1984. *Simone Weil: An Introduction to Her Thought*. Philadelphia: Fortress.

Hillman, James. 1977a. "Inquiry into Image." *Spring*, pp. 62–68.

————. 1977b. *Re-Visioning Psychology*. New York: Harper and Row.

————. 1978. "Further Notes on Images." *Spring*, pp. 152–82.

————. 1979. "Image-Sense." *Spring*, pp. 130–43.

————. 1983. *Healing Fiction*. Barrytown, N.Y.: Station Hill Press.

————. 1985. *Anima: An Anatomy of a Personified Notion*. Dallas: Spring Publications.

————. 1989. *A Blue Fire: Selected Writings by James Hillman*, ed. by Thomas Moore. New York: Harper and Row.

Jones, Richard. 1985. *Poetry and Politics*. New York: William Morrow.

Jung, C. G. 1958. *Psyche and Symbol*, ed. by Violet de Laszlo. New York: Doubleday.

————. 1969. *The Collected Works of C. G. Jung*, trans. by R. F. C. Hull. Bollingen Series XX. Vol. 9, part 1: *The Archetypes and the Collective Unconscious*. Princeton: Princeton University Press.

————. 1969. *The Collected Works of C. G. Jung*, trans. by R. F. C. Hull. Bollingen Series XX. Vol. 8: *The Structure and Dynamics of the Psyche*. Princeton, N.J.: Princeton University Press.

Kaprow, Allan. 1965. *Assemblage, Environments and Happenings*. New York: Harry N. Abrams.

Knill, Paolo. 1978. *Intermodal Learning in Education and Therapy*. Cambridge, Mass.: published by author, 1978.

Kundera, Milan. 1991. *Immortality*, trans. by Peter Kussi. New York: Grove Weidenfeld.

Landgarten, Helen, and Darcy Lubbers. 1991. *Adult Art Psychotherapy*. New York: Brunner/Mazel.

Lawrence, D. H. 1950. *Women in Love* (1920). New York: Viking Press.

―――――. 1953. *St. Mawr* and *The Man Who Died*. New York: Vintage Books.

―――――. 1972. *Studies in Classic American Literature* (1923). New York: Viking Press.

―――――. 1986. *Fantasia of the Unconscious* (1922) and *Psychoanalysis and the Unconscious* (1921). New York: Penguin Books.

McNiff, Shaun. 1973. "A New Perspective in Group Art Therapy." *Art Psychotherapy* 1: 3–4.

―――――. 1974a. *Art Therapy at Danvers*. Andover: Addison Gallery of American Art.

―――――. 1974b. "Organizing Visual Perception through Art." *Academic Therapy* 9: 6.

―――――. 1977. "Motivation in Art." *Art Psychotherapy* 4: 3–4.

―――――. 1981. *The Arts and Psychotherapy*. Springfield, Ill.: Charles C. Thomas.

―――――. 1986a. *Educating the Creative Arts Therapist: A Profile of the Profession*. Springfield, Ill.: Charles C. Thomas.

―――――. 1986b. *Fundamentals of Art Therapy*. Springfield, Ill.: Charles C. Thomas.

―――――. 1989. *Depth Psychology of Art*. Springfield, Ill.: Charles C. Thomas.

Melville, Herman. 1961. *Moby Dick* (1851). New York: New American Library.

Moon, Bruce. 1990. *Existential Art Therapy: The Canvas Mirror*. Springfield, Ill.: Charles C. Thomas.

Moore, Thomas. 1990. *Dark Eros: The Imagination of Sadism*. Dallas: Spring Publications.

Nietzsche, Friedrich. 1917. *Thus Spake Zarathustra*, tran. by Thomas Common. New York: Boni and Liveright.

―――――. 1967. *The Birth of Tragedy* (1872) and *The Case of Wagner* (1888), trans. by Walter Kaufmann. New York: Vintage Press.

Prinzhorn, Hans. 1932. *Psychotherapy: Its Nature, Assumptions, Limitations* (1929), trans. by A. Eiloart. London: Jonathan Cape.

―――――. 1972. *The Artistry of the Mentally Ill* (1922). New York: Springer-Verlag.

Rank, Otto. 1968. *Art and Artists*. New York: Agathon.

Rexine, John. 1985. "*Daimon* in Classical Greek Literature." *Greek Orthodox Theological Review* 30:3, 335–61.

Rubin, William. 1968. *Dada, Surrealism, and Their Heritage*. New York: Museum of Modern Art.

Sandrow, Nahma. 1972. *Surrealism: Theater, Arts, Ideas*. New York: Harper and Row.

Stanislavski, Constantin. 1972. *An Actor Prepares* (1936), trans. by Elizabeth Reynolds Hapgood. New York: Theatre Arts Books.

Suzuki, Shunryu. 1970. *Zen Mind, Beginner's Mind*, ed. by Trudy Dixon. New York and Tokyo: Weatherhill.

Temin, Christine. 1991. "A Little Museum with a Mission." *Boston Globe*, January 2.

Tripp, Edward. 1970. *Crowell's Handbook of Classical Mythology*. New York: Thomas Crowell.

Walker, Barbara. 1983. *The Woman's Encyclopedia of Myths and Secrets*. San Francisco: Harper and Row.

Watkins, Mary. 1983. "The Characters Speak Because They Want to Speak." *Spring*, pp. 13–33.

_____. 1986. *Invisible Guests: The Development of Imaginal Dialogues*. Hillsdale, N.J.: Analytic Press.

Whitman, Walt. 1926. *Leaves of Grass* (1891). Garden City, N.Y.: Doubleday.

Yeats, W. B. 1955. *Collected Poems of W. B. Yeats*. London: Macmillan.

Index